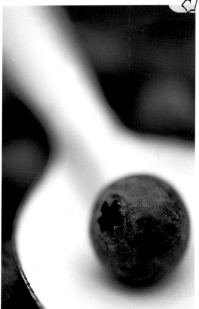

Wonderfoods

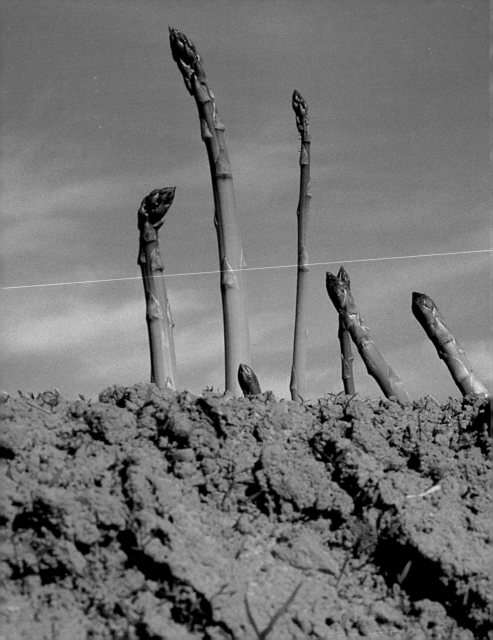

Wonderfoods

Natalie Savona

photographs by Jill Mead

Quadrille

Dedication

This book is dedicated to those who have the privilege of choosing and producing wonderfoods, that they enjoy doing so and that they support those who do not have that choice.

Notes

Each wonderfood chapter is color coded, as you will see from the contents list opposite. However many wonderfoods benefit several systems or areas of the body. The color bars alongside the text introducing each wonderfood highlight other relevant areas.

All recipes serve 4 unless otherwise stated.

I recommend you use fresh herbs, coarse sea or kosher salt, and freshly ground black pepper, unless otherwise suggested.

I use large eggs—ideally organic, otherwise free-range. I also recommend that you buy organic poultry.

Timings are for convection ovens. If you are using a traditional oven, increase the temperature by about 50°F. Use an oven thermometer to check the temperature.

The statements made in this book have not been evaluated by the Food and Drug Administration. The foods and recipes described in this book are not intended to diagnose, treat, cure, or prevent any disease.

Editorial director **Anne Furniss**
Creative director **Helen Lewis**
Project editors **Janet Illsley, Norma MacMillan**
Senior designer **Ros Holder**
Photographer **Jill Mead**
Production **Ruth Deary**

This edition first published in 2007 by Quadrille Publishing

Reprinted in 2008
10 9 8 7 6 5 4 3 2

Text © 2006 **Natalie Savona**
Photography © 2006 **Jill Mead**
Design and layout © 2006
Quadrille Publishing Limited

ISBN-13: 978 184400 476 8

Printed and bound in Singapore

Library of Congress Cataloging-in-Publication Data

Savona, Natalie.
  Wonderfoods : amazing ingredients and recipes for optimum health / Natalie
Savona ; photographs by Jill Mead.
      p. cm.
  Includes index.
  ISBN 978-1-84400-476-8 (pbk.)
  1. Functional foods. 2. Large type books. I. Title.
QP144.F85S28 2008
  613.2--dc22

2008002952

introduction

It is possible to thrive solely on the wonderfoods described in this book. Well, you'd need one addition for your health—water —and perhaps others every now and then for your soul, like cheesecake or coffee, but, by and large, wonderfoods are abundant, easy to get hold of, and remarkably delicious. Even if not all are to your taste, many will be and you may even surprise yourself by starting to like new ones.

Pretty much all foods in their natural state would qualify as wonderfoods. Whoever designed them all did a very good job in packing them with what we need for fit, well bodies that will last us healthily into old age. The trouble is that we get diverted somewhere along the way to foods that challenge our bodies—ones that have been "refined" to make them more appealing, a process that invariably takes some of the goodness away. Refined foods generally have sugar, fat, salt, and chemicals added to them to make them taste "better," or preserve them for longer.

There's certainly no harm in having such foods occasionally —a good-quality pizza, a few glasses of wine, and some ice cream are surely a good way to share food. But when such foods make up the majority of our diet—say, after a day of toast and jelly, cookies, ham sandwich and potato chips, fizzy drink, an apple, a chocolate bar—we become hooked. Even the seemingly healthier options, like a tuna sandwich or rice crackers instead of chips, are often smothered in mayonnaise and salt. After such salty, sweet, fatty foods, a mound of steamed, green vegetables, plain broiled meat, and brown rice seem boring to our palates and to our minds.

If you're reading this book, you're either already cherishing the deliciousness and goodness of wonderfoods, or you are prepared to be inspired by them. You'll find you could fill your shopping cart just with wonderfoods and still not have bought two-thirds of those available.

Not all wonderfoods are necessarily wonderful for you though. Each of us is individual in terms of our nutritional needs and health conditions, not to mention our tastes. While a tomato, for example, is a rich source of the powerful antioxidants vitamin C and lycopene, for someone with arthritis this may trigger joint pain. Raw foods are always touted as wonderfully healthy and energizing. Yet for a weak digestive system, raw food and whole grains are hard work. Although fruits are indisputably wonderfoods, in large amounts they can upset blood sugar and energy levels, and cause bloating. Most of us know what suits us and what doesn't; if you're not sure, it's best to consult a health professional to help you work out your ideal diet.

Selecting the entries for this wonderfoods book was easy enough—virtually all fruit and vegetables, herbs, whole grains, nuts, seeds, and quality proteins qualify. The difficulty was whittling them down to fit into a reasonably sized book! At this stage, it became somewhat random—"If we have broccoli, kale, and cabbage, then perhaps the less popular Brussels sprout will have to go!" Then came the categorization. This, too, took on a somewhat random turn after I'd listed all the things that each food was good for. Many wonderfoods fit into many categories. The color bars alongside the information on each wonderfood guide you to other relevant categories—the contents list on page 6 provides the color key. Garlic, for example, is in the Heart section, but it is also a good Immune and Detox food.

What didn't get into the book were "extras" that you might add to foods, ingredients from healthfood stores, such as wheatgerm, spirulina, or brewers' yeast. All wonderful in themselves, but not quite foods as such ...

Choosing your wonderfoods
Simply choosing to base your diet on wonderfoods is, in itself, a positive step. A good but very general guide on choosing your foods is this: If a food requires a label to tell you what is in it, think again about buying it. Even supermarkets sell most wonderfoods. On many levels, however, I prefer to buy my food

at smaller places, such as local farm shops, independent healthfood stores, and farmers' markets whenever possible. Eating locally grown, seasonal food should be a priority, though of course it isn't always available. After all, I love brown rice and pineapples, which I would never eat if I only bought my own locally grown produce!

From the point of view of chemicals used in growing food, organic produce is always the best choice. Even just a couple of organic items in your weekly shop is useful in helping to minimize your chemical exposure. But two points here: There is a good argument for choosing locally grown, non-organic food over organic varieties flown halfway across the world that has possibly been farmed by underpaid workers. Secondly, just because something is organic, it doesn't mean it's good for you —organic cake and coffee with organic milk and sugar is still a big hit on the sugar and stimulant front.

Preparing your wonderfoods
The recipes I have created here make use of as many wonderfoods as I could cram into each one and, you'll find, they are largely very simple to prepare. Even the recipes with longer lists of ingredients usually require only one pan or dish and very little effort.

You can rustle up a wonderfully tasty meal with just a few fresh ingredients as long as you keep a good stock of pantry and refrigerator essentials, such as paprika, cayenne pepper, Chinese five spice, olives, peppercorns in a mill, a jar of tahini, garlic, bouillon powder such as Marigold, tamari (a type of soy sauce), hot pepper sauce, Thai curry paste, miso paste, balsamic vinegar, cans of beans and chickpeas, cans of tomatoes, plenty of brown rice, oats, and other grains, nuts, and seeds.

A word about fats & sugar

I generally suggest using light olive oil for cooking as it is a monounsaturated fat. This means that it is chemically less susceptible to the damage from heat that affects sunflower and other seed oils, turning them into harmful trans fats. When you are softening onions or stir-frying, I recommend a method called "steam-frying," which is pretty much the same thing, but you use less oil and add a little water to stop burning or sticking. Butter does give a particular flavor to some recipes, but because it is high in saturated fat, it is best used sparingly, just for flavor. Blending it with olive oil also helps prevent it from burning.

Some recipes call for sugar. I think that, used sparingly, sugar is a perfectly reasonable part of a varied, healthy diet. Honey, maple syrup, and molasses offer not only a different flavor from sugar, but also a different nutrient base, although they are still, essentially, sugars. For this reason they are not valid substitutes for anyone who is avoiding sugar, such as a diabetic. One sugar substitute that I use very occasionally is xylitol, which sounds very chemical-like, but is a natural product extracted from plants. It looks and tastes like sugar, but does not raise blood-sugar levels in the same way, is lower in calories, and helps prevent tooth decay.

My "thing" on food

I was recently asked what my "thing" was about food, what philosophy I espouse. And I'm often asked, "Do you believe in x, y, or z?" regarding specific ways of eating, such as veganism, raw food diet, high protein diet, or whatever.

My "thing" is to ensure that you eat a broad range of good-quality foods and to enjoy what you eat. Do this, while being sensitive to what really works for you as an individual and that doesn't just mean for instant gratification. Just because your body is crying out for doughnuts every day at 11am, it doesn't mean they must be right for you. That said, I've seen far too many health-obsessed people control their diet to such a degree that the rigidity makes them irritable and ill, and the odd doughnut would probably do them good. After all, there's no point worrying so much about whether a food contains a little sugar if the worrying itself is going to give you an ulcer!

Food—preparing and sharing it—is, for those of us privileged to have the choice, one of life's joys, and if you base what you eat on wonderfoods, you can't really go wrong.

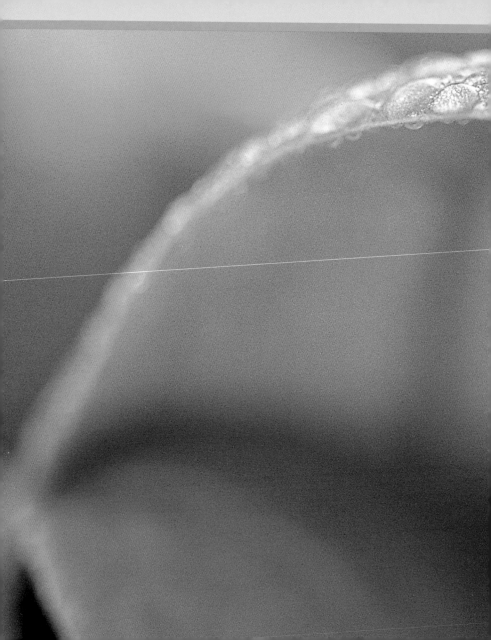

energy

The wonderfoods in this section are, indeed, packed with nutrients, starch, and sweetness, which translate as energy that you can harness. They are of a variety that will leave you satisfied and, at the same time, provide you with good doses of important micronutrients—vitamins, minerals, and other substances that are needed for countless uses in the body. The sure-fire way of getting an instant hit of energy is to have a strong, sugary coffee or some candy—that is, if you also want a sure way of crashing soon afterward, setting up a vicious cycle of energy boost and exhaustion.

The body digests the sugars and starches within energy foods into sugar molecules that can be released into the bloodstream. The sugar is then carried around the body to cells, where it is used to make energy. Quick-fix energy-giving foods, such as candy, or those made with refined (white) flour, are rapidly digested and released into the bloodstream as sugar soon after eating. Although this may seem like a good idea in the short-term, what goes up must come down. The body quickly responds to reduce rising blood-sugar levels, so you then feel a crash in energy, as well as in mood and concentration. The one thing that goes back up is your appetite...for another quick fix.

By contrast, energizing wonderfoods contain fiber, fat, vitamins, and minerals, which help regulate the rate at which they are converted into energy. So you still get a lift, but in a much more even, sustained way. You also get the vitamins and minerals that are involved in the actual conversion process to energy and other tasks around the body.

If you are consistently low in energy, you need to look at the whole of your diet, not just significantly boost your intake of the energy wonderfoods. You could try: making sure you have breakfast and evenly spaced meals throughout the day; not relying on quick fixes such as coffee, which are false friends; eating a variety of wonderfoods at each meal, such as a banana with yogurt and pumpkin seeds for breakfast, or sweet potato with chicken and broccoli for dinner.

You also need to ascertain and deal with the triggers for your tiredness. Insufficient sleep (obvious, but remarkably common), reliance on quick hits, low iron stores (common in vegetarians or vegans), over- or under-exercizing, sluggish digestion, and low moods can be causes of long-term fatigue. Whatever is going on for you, incorporating the wonderfoods in this chapter, alongside others in the book, can go a long way to energizing you.

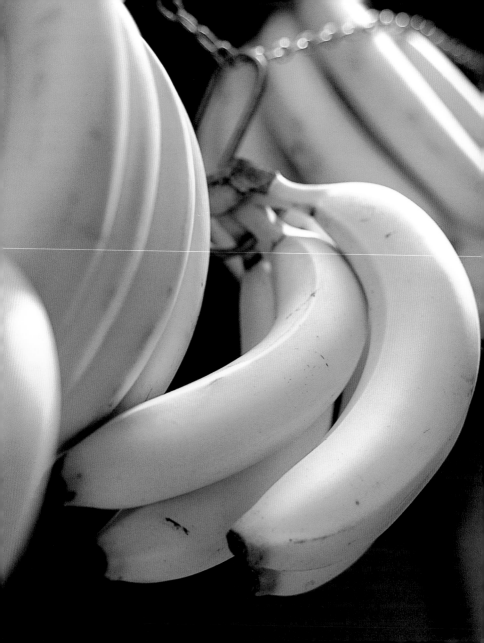

banana

Perhaps the ultimate fast food, bananas are understandably one of the most popular energy-boosters. A ripe banana is easy to digest, as most of the starch has been converted to sugar, and can help relieve constipation (unripe ones may cause it). It is sugar combined with fiber that makes bananas so good for a sustained release of energy, even more so if eaten with some nuts or yogurt. Fructo-oligo-saccharides (FOS) in bananas help feed "good bacteria" in the gut. The pectin fiber in the fruit helps to soothe heartburn, ulcers, or inflammation in the digestive tract, and to lower cholesterol. Bananas are also a good source of vitamin B_6 and, like all fruits and vegetables, contain the mineral potassium. They also contain tryptophan, which the body can convert to serotonin—a hormone that helps lift moods and promote sleep. Multinational corporations cultivate vast swathes of former rainforest in Central and South America to produce cheap bananas, so buy Fair Trade bananas to support fairer, smaller producers.

almond baked bananas

A COMFORTING DESSERT THAT COMBINES COMPLEMENTARY TASTES AND TEXTURES. USE BANANAS THAT ARE RIPE BUT FIRM.

4 **bananas**, peeled and sliced lengthwise
8 **strawberries**, washed, hulled, and halved
juice of 2 **oranges**
generous splash of amaretto liqueur
$^1/_2$ tbsp butter
2$^1/_2$ tbsp chopped **almonds**
plain **yogurt** for serving

Preheat the oven to 350°F. Lay the bananas and strawberries in a baking dish. Pour the orange juice and amaretto over the fruit and dot with the butter. Sprinkle on the almonds and bake until the bananas are soft, 15–20 minutes.

Serve topped with a dollop of yogurt.

frozen coco-nana

FROZEN BANANAS ALONE ARE LIKE AN ICE CREAM TREAT, BUT THIS COMBINATION MAKES THEM EVEN BETTER.

4 **bananas**, peeled
1 heaped tbsp shredded
   coconut (ideally fresh,
   otherwise use dried)
1 heaped tbsp **sesame seeds**
½ cup **coconut** milk
1 tbsp **honey**
juice of 1 **lime**
splash of rum (optional)

Chop the bananas into 1-inch pieces, lay them on a metal tray, and put them in the freezer for at least an hour.

In a dry frying pan, toast the shredded coconut and sesame seeds until golden brown.

Just before serving, get the bananas out of the freezer and whiz in a blender with the coconut milk, honey, and lime juice until smooth, adding a splash of rum, if desired.

Spoon into small serving bowls, top with the toasted coconut and sesame seeds, and serve.

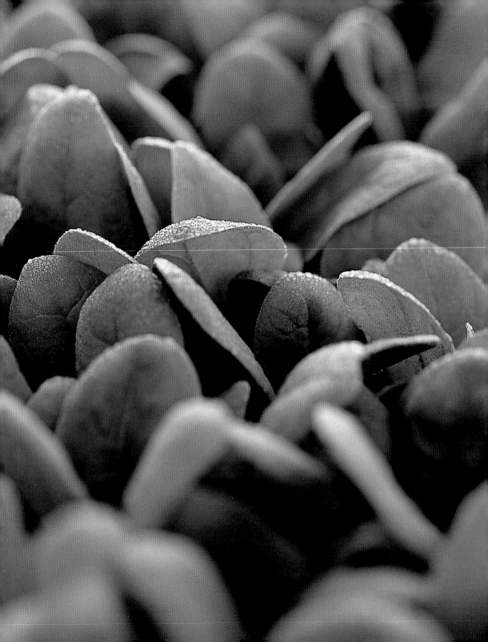

spinach

Spinach is perhaps best known for its iron content, thanks to Popeye, although the iron in spinach is not in its most accessible form to humans (compared with meat, for example). Despite this, it is a godsend for vegetarians and vegans, and a squeeze of lemon juice will provide vitamin C, which helps iron absorption. Iron is essential for healthy blood cells, enabling them to carry oxygen efficiently around the body for every cell to create energy—one of the first signs of being low in iron is fatigue. Spinach is also laden with other important nutrients, such as calcium (150% more than milk, weight for weight), magnesium (a mineral that a great many women are low in), and beta-carotene, the vegetable form of vitamin A and a useful antioxidant. A substance called neoxanthin in spinach has been shown to help prostate health. Vitamin K, also contained in spinach, is important for bone health and blood clotting. The green in leaves, including spinach, comes from the chlorophyll, a substance that, along with the fiber, acts as a powerful "cleanser."

spinach tart

EVEN PEOPLE WHO AREN'T BIG FANS OF GREEN VEGGIES USUALLY LOVE THIS
CLASSIC RECIPE. LEFTOVERS, IF THERE ARE ANY, ARE IDEAL FOR A PACKED LUNCH
OR PICNIC. *SERVES 2*

1 tbsp olive oil, plus extra
  for brushing
2 medium **onions**, peeled
  and finely chopped
2 **garlic** cloves, peeled
  and crushed
10 oz **spinach**, washed
  and chopped
about 20 olives, pitted
  and chopped
1 heaped tbsp finely
  chopped mint
1 heaped tbsp finely
  chopped **parsley**
1 **egg**, beaten
7 oz feta cheese, finely
  crumbled
1 heaped tbsp **sunflower
  seeds**
8 sheets of phyllo pastry

Preheat the oven to 350°F. Heat the olive oil in
a frying pan, add the onions and garlic, and cook
over low heat for about 5 minutes to soften. Add
the spinach and stir until it has wilted, then tip
into a large bowl. Add the olives, herbs, egg, feta,
and sunflower seeds, and toss to mix.

Layer the phyllo sheets in a 10-inch tart pan,
leaving some overhanging the rim all around and
brushing each layer with olive oil. Pour the filling
into the phyllo shell and roughly crumple the
overhanging pastry back up to edge the tart. Bake
until the filling is set and the phyllo is golden
brown, 30–35 minutes.

duck & spinach salad

THIS MAKES A SUPERB LUNCH OR SUMMER SUPPER—ONE TO IMPRESS GUESTS.
YOU COULD USE PAPAYA INSTEAD OF THE MANGO.

*4 boneless duck breast
halves, with skin
2 heaped tsp Chinese five
spice powder
sprinkling of cayenne
pepper
8 oz baby **spinach** leaves,
washed
1 **mango**, peeled, pitted,
and diced
handful of cilantro leaves,
roughly chopped
4 **scallions**, trimmed
and sliced
2 large, cooked **beets**,
peeled and diced
1/3 English **cucumber**,
chopped
juice of 1 **lime**
1 1/2 tbsp tamari or soy sauce
2 tbsp toasted **sesame** oil*

Preheat the oven to 350°F. Score the skin side of each duck breast a few times and rub with the Chinese five spice and cayenne pepper, pushing some into the slashes to touch the meat.

Preheat a dry frying pan and quickly fry the duck, skin down, for about 5 minutes. Turn the duck breasts and fry for a couple of minutes longer, then place in a baking dish and finish cooking in the oven for about 10 minutes, depending on how pink you like your meat and how thick the breasts are. Let rest in a warm place for 5 minutes.

Meanwhile, in a large bowl, toss the spinach with all the other ingredients, then divide among plates. Slice each duck breast and arrange on top. Serve at once, while the duck is still warm.

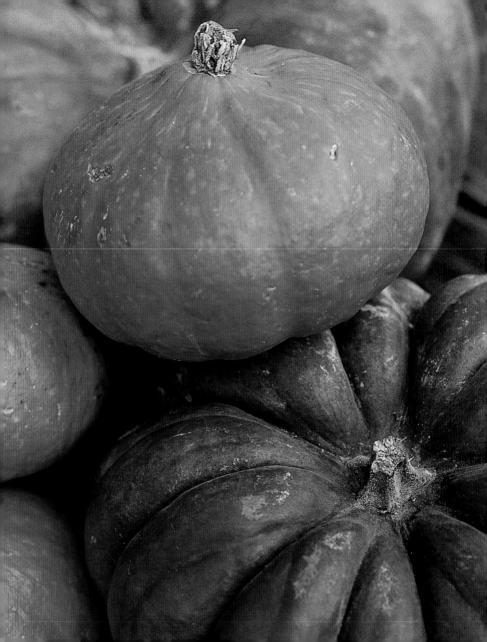

winter
squash

Native to the Americas, where it was originally used to make flour, the lowly pumpkin may be what got the Pilgrims through their first winter in 1620. For those who count, pumpkin is remarkably low in calories, although its starch is good for energy. It was used as a folk remedy to kill intestinal worms, the seeds being more effective than the flesh. Pumpkin is high in fiber, which is useful for easing food through the intestines and helping clear waste. As its orange color suggests, pumpkin contains beta-carotene, which, among other things, helps protect against the harmful rays of the sun. Apart from pumpkins, the family of winter squashes comes in a wide variety of shapes, sizes, and colors, perhaps the most tasty being the butternut. All winter squashes can be roasted, boiled and mashed, used in soups, stews, savory and sweet pies, and breads, and even grated to eat raw. Because pumpkin can be bland, many recipes add heaps of fat or sugar, but steer clear of those to get the gains from this versatile, filling vegetable.

butternut & feta salad

FRESH, RAW SPINACH OFFSETS COMFORTING WARM SQUASH AND CRUMBLY FETA CHEESE PERFECTLY. SERVE THIS SALAD AS A SUBSTANTIAL LUNCH OR LIGHT DINNER.

1 small butternut **squash**, roughly cubed

1 red **bell pepper**, cored, seeded, and cut into squares

few **thyme** sprigs, or 1/2 tsp dried thyme

splash of olive oil

dash of balsamic vinegar

freshly ground black pepper

8 oz baby **spinach** leaves, washed

3 **scallions**, trimmed and finely sliced

squeeze of **lemon** juice

8–12 cherry **tomatoes**, quartered

7 oz feta cheese, cubed

Preheat the oven to 350°F. Don't bother to peel the squash for this, but do scoop out the seeds. Put it into a roasting pan with the red pepper and thyme, plus generous dashes of olive oil and balsamic vinegar. Season with pepper and toss well. Roast for about 40 minutes.

Meanwhile, pile the spinach equally on four plates. Scatter the scallions over, drizzle with a little olive oil, and add a squeeze of lemon juice.

When the squash and red pepper are cooked, let them cool slightly, then mix in the tomatoes and feta. Pile the warm mixture on top of the spinach leaves and eat immediately. Delicious with warm, crusty brown rolls.

pumpkin & bacon soup

BACON MAY NOT BE THE HEALTHIEST OF FOODS, BUT ITS SALTINESS COMBINED WITH RATHER BLAND, SWEET PUMPKIN IS DELICIOUS. EATEN WITH WHOLE-WHEAT BREAD, THIS SOUP MAKES A SATISFYING MEAL IN ITSELF, OR YOU CAN SERVE IT AS A WARMING APPETIZER BEFORE A LIGHT MAIN COURSE.

*1 large wedge of **pumpkin**, or 1 large butternut **squash***
*1 large **onion**, peeled and finely diced*
*2 **celery** stalks, sliced*
a little olive oil
12–14 oz slab bacon or smoked ham, diced
freshly ground black pepper
4 cups vegetable or chicken stock
*handful of **parsley**, chopped*

Peel the pumpkin or squash, remove seeds, and cut into cubes. (The soup will be even sweeter and richer if you roast the pumpkin at this stage for 30 minutes at 350°F, but it's not essential.)

In a large, covered saucepan over low heat, soften the onion with the celery in a little olive oil. Add the bacon and cook, stirring, for a few minutes until evenly colored.

Add the pumpkin, season with pepper, and then pour in the stock. Simmer, covered, until the pumpkin is soft, about 30 minutes depending on the variety (or much less if pre-roasted).

Whiz the soup briefly using an immersion blender, to purée some of the pumpkin and thicken the liquid, but keeping a chunky texture. Stir in the chopped parsley and serve.

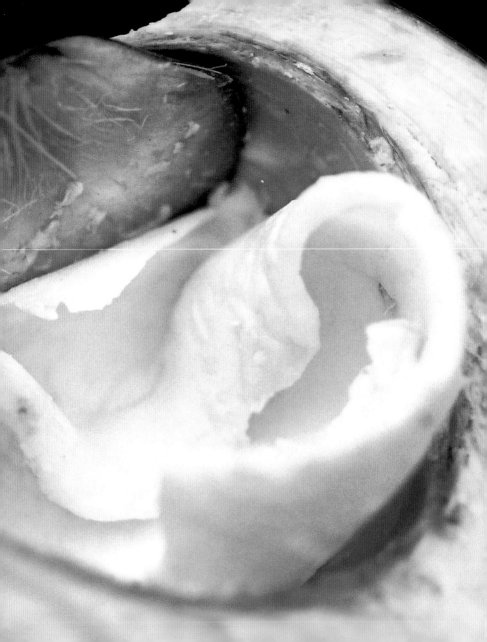

coconut

In India, coconut palms are considered a *kalpavriksha*, or tree of life, and, indeed, pretty much every part of the plant is used. Although coconuts are one of the rare sources of saturated fat (SF) in plants, it's not all bad news. About half of a coconut's saturated fats are known as "medium chain triglycerides," or MCTs, which seem to increase the burning of calories, i.e. they promote energy production and are not stored in the body as fat. So it seems coconut can actually help boost energy and weight loss. MCTs are also easily digested and absorbed, unlike other saturated fats. Coconuts are a rich source of an MCT called lauric acid (as is breast milk), which the body can convert into an antiviral and antibacterial substance called monolaurin. They also contain a little of the antifungal caprylic acid. Because it is high in SF, coconut oil is, like butter, good for cooking, as it is not denatured by heat. But like all fatty foods, coconut should be eaten in moderation.

aromatic fish packets

I FIRST TASTED THIS WHEN MY FRIEND, CHARMAINE, COOKED IT FOR DINNER ON A WINTER'S NIGHT IN A THATCHED FARMHOUSE IN ENGLAND. NOT VERY TRADITIONAL, BUT WARMING ALL THE SAME, ESPECIALLY WHEN SERVED WITH BROWN RICE AND STIR-FRIED VEGETABLES.

4 **fish** fillets, such as
    haddock or snapper
2 lemongrass stalks, sliced
2 **garlic** cloves, peeled and
    sliced
1-inch piece fresh **ginger**,
    peeled and sliced
1 fresh, hot chile, seeded
    and finely sliced (more if
    you like it hot)
2 **limes**, halved
1 small can **coconut** milk

Preheat the oven to 350°F. Cut four large pieces of parchment paper and fold each one in half—folded, they need to be big enough to enclose a fish fillet with enough paper to scrunch up over the top to seal.

Lay a fish fillet in the middle of each doubled piece of paper. Scatter the lemongrass, garlic, ginger, and chile over and under the fish fillets and squeeze the juice of $1/2$ lime over each one. Fold up the sides of the paper, then drizzle about 2 tbsp coconut milk on each fillet.

Bring the edges of the paper together over the fish, then roll and scrunch them together, tucking in the ends to form little packets. Place on a baking sheet and bake for about 15 minutes, depending on the thickness of the fillets.

Serve the fish in their paper packets on warm plates, with stir-fried vegetables and brown rice.

mango with coconut rice

DURING APRIL IN THAILAND, STALLS AT THE SIDE OF THE ROAD ARE PILED HIGH
WITH RIPE MANGOES…IT'S HARD TO RESIST HAVING SERVING AFTER SERVING OF
THIS DELICIOUS, RICH MANGO AND RICE DISH.

3/4 cup **brown rice** (or Thai
fragrant rice)
1 heaped tbsp **sesame seeds**
1 cup **coconut** milk
3 tbsp sugar or alternative
equivalent (see page 10)
2 ripe **mangoes**, peeled and
sliced off the pit

Cook the rice according to the package directions.

Meanwhile, in a dry frying pan over moderate heat, toss the sesame seeds until they start to pop. Set aside to cool.

When the rice is cooked, drain if necessary, then add the coconut milk and sugar and stir over the heat until you have a thick mass of rice that's sticky but not runny, about 10 minutes.

Let the rice cool a little before serving in small bowls, topped with slices of fresh mango and sprinkled with the toasted sesame seeds.

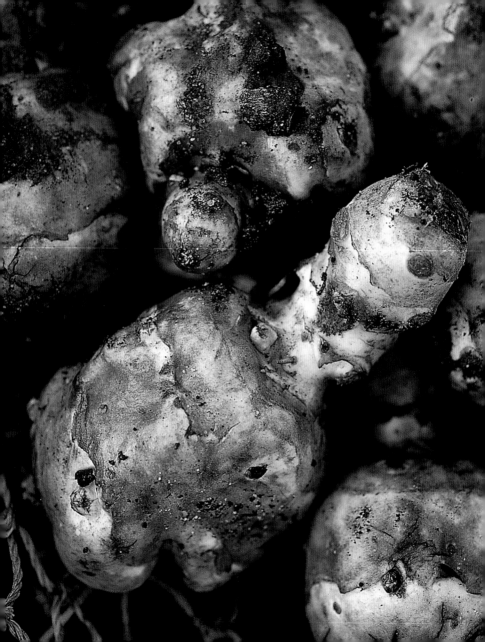

jerusalem artichoke

Jerusalem artichokes are not remotely related to the more familiar globe artichokes and they have nothing to do with Jerusalem. In fact, they are a member of the sunflower family and are sometimes called sunchokes. The tubers have a delicate, nutty flavor and can be used similarly to potatoes: boiled, steamed, mashed, in soups, baked, or fried, but also raw. Unlike potatoes, sunchokes provide a gentle release of their energy, because they store it as inulin rather than sugar. So they are a good food for people with diabetes or poor blood-sugar balance. It is the soluble fiber, inulin, that gives them their notoriety for inducing wind, because it is a "prebiotic," i.e. it feeds the good bacteria in the gut. A plus point is that inulin can bind with waste products or toxins, helping to escort them out of the body. Studies have shown that inulin can help to lower cholesterol levels, too. Jerusalem artichokes also contain good amounts of iron—weight for weight, even more than lean beef.

jerusalem chicken

THIS A BEAUTIFULLY FLAVORED DISH FROM THE MIDDLE EAST. ALTHOUGH THE NAME OF THE VEGETABLE SUGGESTS THAT IT ORIGINATES FROM THIS REGION, IT IS NATIVE TO NORTH AMERICA AND RELATED TO THE SUNFLOWER. JERUSALEM ARTICHOKE IS THOUGHT TO BE A CORRUPTION OF *GIRASOLE*, THE ITALIAN WORD FOR SUNFLOWER, MEANING "TURNING TO THE SUN."

2 tbsp olive oil
4 tbsp **lemon** juice
10 **garlic** cloves, peeled and halved
7 oz **Jerusalem artichokes,** peeled and sliced
10 **cardamom** pods
6 saffron threads (or ½ tsp ground **turmeric**)
freshly ground black pepper
8 **chicken** thighs (or drumsticks, if you prefer)
12–15 **basil** leaves
2 heaped tbsp pine nuts, lightly toasted

In a large saucepan, mix the olive oil and lemon juice, then add the garlic, Jerusalem artichokes, cardamom, saffron, and some pepper. Add enough water to cover the artichokes and bring to a boil. Add the chicken pieces and stir, then cover and simmer gently for an hour.

Just before serving, stir in the basil leaves and scatter the pine nuts over. Serve with brown rice and a steamed green vegetable, such as spinach.

jerusalem artichoke bake

THIS IS A SLIGHTLY HEALTHIER VERSION OF THE TRADITIONAL DAUPHINOISE,
WHICH IS USUALLY MADE WITH POTATOES AND LOTS OF CREAM. IT GOES WELL
WITH ANY MEAT OR CHICKEN DISH.

10 oz **Jerusalem artichokes**,
  well scrubbed and
  thinly sliced
10 oz celeriac, peeled and
  thinly sliced
1 **onion**, peeled and
  finely sliced
1 **garlic** clove, peeled
  and crushed
1 cup vegetable or chicken
  stock
1 cup sour cream
freshly ground black pepper
pinch of freshly grated
  nutmeg
1 **egg**
handful of grated Gruyère
  cheese

Preheat the oven to 350°F. Layer the Jerusalem
artichokes, celeriac, and onion in a shallow baking
dish, sprinkling with the garlic.

Mix the stock with the sour cream, season
with pepper and nutmeg, and beat in the egg.
Gently pour this mixture over the vegetables and
top with the cheese. Bake for about 40 minutes,
checking whether the vegetables are cooked
through after about 30 minutes by poking a
skewer into the middle.

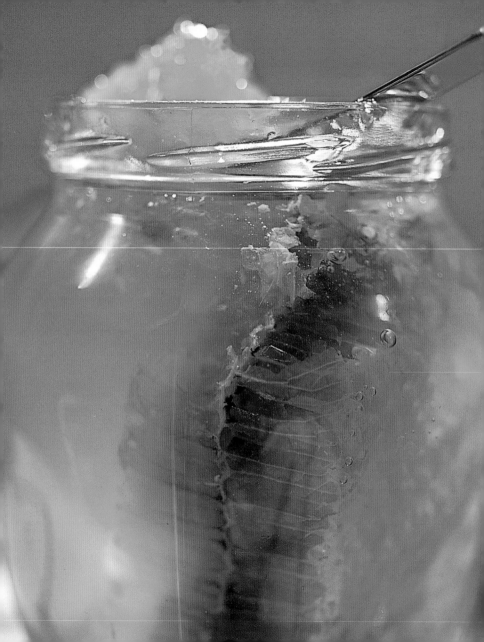

honey

Reputed to be the food of the gods, honey has even crept into our language to mean love. It is 97% sugar and primarily a source of energy that is easily absorbed by the body. For this reason, it shouldn't be used excessively or on its own, otherwise it contributes to tooth decay, weight gain, and even diabetes. To get more than just a unique sweetener—and the best of that remaining 3%—it's essential to eat raw honey, harvested by scrupulous beekeepers who do not allow medication or sugar to contaminate their product. The qualities of the honey also depend on the flowers from which the nectar came—for example, manuka honey from New Zealand has the antiseptic properties of the manuka tree. Raw honey contains residues of propolis—a resinlike substance made by bees with healing and antimicrobial properties—used for centuries on the skin to treat burns, wounds, and ulcers. Another natural sweetener containing valuable nutrients, especially iron and other minerals, is blackstrap molasses, a byproduct of sugar refining.

honeyed granola

THIS RECIPE MAKES A BIG BATCH OF CEREAL THAT CAN BE STORED IN A SEALED CONTAINER FOR A MONTH OR SO. *MAKES 10–12 SERVINGS*

6¼ cups rolled **oats**

2 heaped tbsp **sunflower seeds**

2 heaped tbsp **pumpkin seeds**

2 heaped tbsp **almonds** or hazelnuts, roughly broken

2 heaped tbsp dried shredded **coconut**

½ cup **honey**

½ cup **coconut** oil or olive oil

2 tsp vanilla extract

3 heaped tbsp raisins or dried cranberries

8 dried **apricots**, finely chopped

Preheat the oven to 325°F. Line a large, shallow baking pan with parchment paper.

In a large bowl, combine the oats, seeds, nuts, and coconut. In a small saucepan, heat the honey, oil, and vanilla extract. Just before the mixture boils, pour it over the dry ingredients and mix well.

Spread out the mixture in the prepared pan and bake for about 25 minutes, stirring it halfway through cooking. As soon as you take it out of the oven, add the dried fruit and toss to mix.

Let the granola cool completely before storing it in an airtight container. Eat a bowlful for breakfast, with milk or soymilk.

honey-broiled salmon

THIS HAS A LOVELY SMOKY FLAVOR (YOU COULD ALSO GRILL THE SALMON). THE
MARINADE WORKS WELL ON CHICKEN OR LAMB, TOO.

*4 fresh **salmon** steaks
   or fillets*
FOR THE MARINADE
*2 tbsp **honey***
1 tsp smoked paprika
$1/2$ tsp hot pepper sauce
1 tbsp cider vinegar
2 tsp tamari or soy sauce

Mix the marinade ingredients together in a large
bowl. Add the fish steaks and swish them around
so they are well coated. Let marinate for about
20 minutes.

Preheat the broiler and broil the salmon
steaks, basting frequently with the marinade, until
cooked to your taste. This should take no longer
than 3 minutes each side, depending on the
thickness of the fish. If you are cooking fillets with
skin, broil skin-side up for about 4 minutes, then
turn and cook flesh-side up for 1 minute only.

Serve with a steamed green vegetable, such as
broccoli or kale.

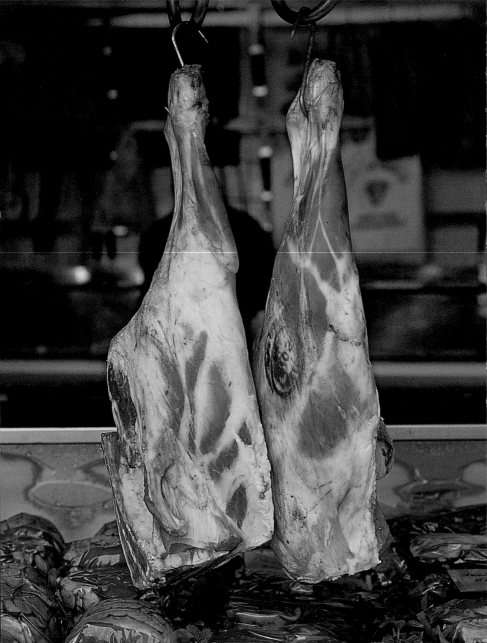

lamb

Red meat is often maligned for its saturated fat and cholesterol. Yes, we should keep those to a minimum, but lean meat such as lamb (or even beef) can be a wonderful addition to a menu. The prime cuts from naturally reared, active animals that graze in fields are generally lean—so you get the goodness with minimal saturated fat and cholesterol. Red meat is an excellent source of protein and easily absorbed iron—more so than any vegetable source of this vital mineral. Iron is fundamental for carrying oxygen throughout the body efficiently, for cells to make energy. Many menstruating women end up low in iron, so eating red meat, such as lamb, is a useful way of avoiding this. Energy-wise, a protein-rich meal is more sustaining, and lamb is also rich in B vitamins, used for, among countless other things, making energy inside our cells. Unlike plant foods, red meat is a particularly good source of vitamin B12, which is needed for good moods and a healthy heart.

lamb curry kebabs

YOU COULD APPLY THIS MARINADE TO ANY MEAT, FISH, OR SHRIMP, BUT LAMB TAKES ON ALL THE SPICES PARTICULARLY WELL. FOR OPTIMUM FLAVOR AND FRAGRANCE, USE WHOLE CUMIN AND CORIANDER SEEDS, TOAST THEM IN A DRY FRYING PAN UNTIL THEY RELEASE THEIR AROMA, THEN GRIND TO A POWDER.

2¼ lb lean, boned **lamb** (ideally leg), cubed

FOR THE MARINADE

1 medium **onion**, peeled and finely diced

3 **garlic** cloves, peeled and crushed

1 tbsp olive oil

3 tbsp **lemon** juice

freshly ground black pepper

2 tsp ground cumin

1 tsp ground coriander

1 tsp paprika

2 heaped tbsp grated **coconut** (ideally fresh, otherwise use dried)

3 tbsp plain **yogurt**

FOR SERVING

handful of cilantro leaves

Mix all the marinade ingredients together in a large bowl. Add the meat and stir well to coat all the pieces thoroughly. Let marinate for at least an hour, ideally 4 or 5 hours.

Preheat the broiler or prepare the grill. Thread the meat onto four long skewers. Broil the kebabs 3–4 inches from the heat, or cook on the grill, turning them occasionally, until browned on all sides but still pink in the middle, 10–12 minutes.

Scatter the cilantro over and serve with Scented savory rice (page 67), Apricot salsa (page 175), and a Wonderfoods green salad (page 111).

grilled lamb with minty tomato salsa

IN LATE SUMMER, MAKE A BIG BOWL OF THIS SALSA TO GO WITH GRILLED MEAT. IT'S
A GOOD WAY TO USE UP YOUR HOMEGROWN TOMATOES THAT HAVEN'T RIPENED.

4 **lamb** steaks or chops
FOR THE TOMATO SALSA
3 large, green **tomatoes**,
　　roughly chopped
2 heaped tbsp chopped
　　mint
1 heaped tbsp chopped
　　parsley
1/2 small red **onion**, peeled
　　and very finely chopped
1 small **garlic** clove, peeled
　　and crushed
1 tbsp olive oil
juice of 1/2 **lemon**
freshly ground black pepper

Put all the ingredients for the tomato salsa in a
serving bowl and toss to mix.

Prepare the grill (or preheat the broiler). Cook
the lamb steaks until nicely browned on the
outside but still pink in the middle, or until they
are done to your taste, 3–5 minutes on each side.

Serve with the tomato salsa and Herby sweet
oven fries (page 198).

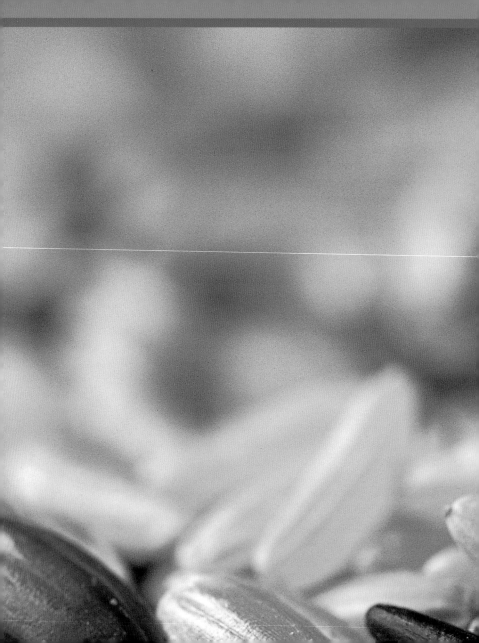

digest

Given that the digestive tract is a long tube comprising different parts, each with their different jobs, there's a long list of essentials for keeping it working efficiently and comfortably. These have to take into account differences between individuals, such as not "going" often enough or "going" too regularly, or those who have a tendency for heartburn and those who can eat anything. The wonderfoods here offer a range of qualities in soothing the gut. It's a matter of finding out what works for you.

One of the most common of all digestive complaints is constipation. This can be tricky to resolve, but the solution may be as simple as eating more vegetables and fruit such as apples. The fiber in these, as in whole grains (such as brown rice and buckwheat), seeds, and legumes, helps bulk out the stool, making it easier to pass. That said, the inherent indigestibility of legumes and the high sugar content of fiber-rich dried fruit make some people bloated and congested—a prime example of our individuality. Another key ingredient for regularity is water, to prevent the stool from becoming dry and impacted in the colon and difficult to pass.

For digestive processes to work smoothly, food needs to be eaten slowly, in manageable quantities and at reasonable intervals. Chewing well and pausing between mouthfuls is the right start. This ensures that the food is mechanically broken down and stimulates the release of digestive juices in the stomach and intestines—gearing the whole system up to process the food well. The more efficiently this happens, the more nutrients you get out of your food and the less likely you are to have digestive difficulties like indigestion or wind. Some foods, such as papaya and pineapple, contain enzymes that actually help the breakdown of food into smaller particles. And spices have been used as digestive aids for many, many years.

Another potential complication with the digestive system is negative reactions to particular foods. There is an increasing awareness that some people do not tolerate certain foods well. Specific foods give them indigestion, bloating, flatulence, constipation, diarrhea, or even symptoms that are seemingly unconnected to the gut, such as lethargy or eczema. Common culprits are wheat (or gluten, which is found not only in wheat, but also in oats, rye, and barley), dairy products, and soy foods. This is a very individual matter that should be explored with a health professional so as not to restrict the diet dangerously or unnecessarily. The wonderfoods in this section are generally fine for most people.

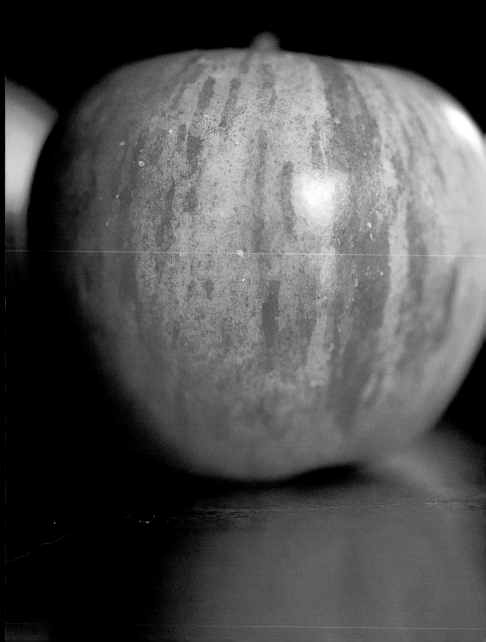

apple

Throughout history, apples have symbolized love and fertility, though it's easy to cast them aside in favor of exotic fruits, especially given the bland taste of many common apples these days. But make careful choices and you cannot do better. Apples contain pectin, a soluble fiber that gently but efficiently cleanses the intestines, binding with waste products and escorting them out of the body. It also encourages the proliferation of beneficial bacteria in the gut, helps keep cholesterol down, and helps balance blood-sugar levels. Apples are a source of quercetin, which helps protect cholesterol from damage that causes a buildup in arteries. They are easily digestible, alkaline, and about 85% water—so are hydrating too. Malic acid is found in apples and this plays a role in all human cells as part of the energy production process. Choosing tasty apples can be hit and miss, so you need to experiment—at farmers' markets and farm shops you are more likely to find unusual, flavorful varieties.

mackerel with apple purée

I FIRST MADE THIS WHEN WE HAD MASSES OF APPLE PURÉE IN THE REFRIGERATOR, PREPARED AFTER PICKING APPLES IN A FRIEND'S ORCHARD. COMBINED WITH THE HORSERADISH, THE PURÉE MAKES A SHARP CONTRAST TO THE OILY FISH.

*2 large, tart cooking **apples**, quartered, cored, and peeled*
*grated zest of 1 **lemon***
3 tbsp water
*4 **mackerel**, cleaned, heads on*
2 heaped tsp horseradish sauce

Roughly chop the cooking apples and put them into a saucepan with the lemon zest and water. Cover and cook slowly until the apples are soft and pulpy.

Preheat the broiler. Score the mackerel two or three times on each side, then cook them under the hot broiler for about 8 minutes, turning halfway through. Really fresh fish can be left slightly underdone.

Mix the horseradish into the warm apple purée. Serve the mackerel with a generous spoonful of spiked apple purée on the side.

apple custard tart

THE INSPIRATION FOR THIS TART IS A COUPLE OF DIFFERENT RECIPES FROM THE WONDERFUL MOOSEWOOD COOKBOOK BY MOLLIE KATZEN. THE BASE HAS A CRUNCHY COARSE TEXTURE. I SOMETIMES MAKE A FINER CRUST BY GRINDING THE OATS IN A BLENDER FOR A MINUTE OR SO BEFORE I START.

FOR THE BASE
1¼ cups rolled **oats**
½ cup chopped hazelnuts
3½ tbsp **sunflower seeds**
1 heaped tbsp brown sugar
    or alternative equivalent
    (see page 10)
pinch of salt
1 tsp ground **cinnamon**
⅓ cup butter, melted

FOR THE FILLING
3 **eggs**
1¼ cups plain **yogurt**
¼ cup brown sugar or
    alternative equivalent
    (see page 10)
2 tsp vanilla extract
1 tsp ground **cinnamon**
2 large, tart cooking **apples**

Preheat the oven to 350°F. For the base, mix the oats, nuts, seeds, sugar, salt, and cinnamon together in a large roasting pan and toast in the oven for about 30 minutes.

Meanwhile, prepare the filling. In a bowl, whisk together the eggs, yogurt, sugar, vanilla extract, and cinnamon. Peel, core, and slice the apples.

Stir the melted butter into the oven-toasted base ingredients, then press the mixture on the bottom of a deep 8-inch tart pan. Lay the sliced apples on the base and carefully pour the filling mixture over them. Bake until golden and firm, 35–40 minutes.

The tart is delicious eaten hot with sour cream or plain yogurt, but it's also good cold.

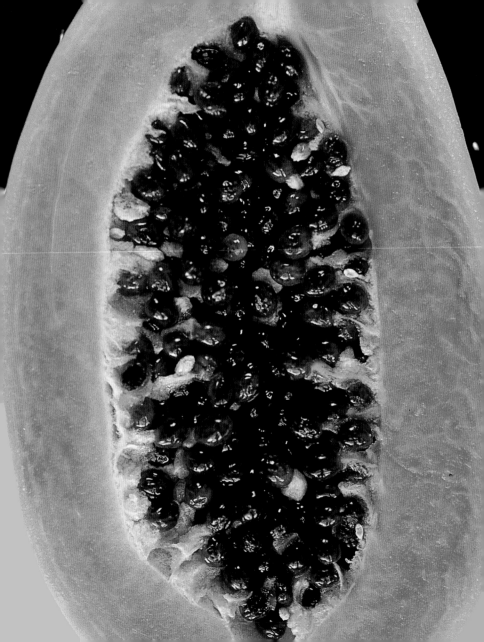

papaya

This fruit is known as *fruta bomba* to polite Cubans because "papaya" is slang in their country for the female sexual organs! The buttery, soft flesh is most often eaten when it is ripe and orange-colored, but it is also popular in savory meals when unripe, hard, and green, as in one of my favorite dishes in the world, Thai som tam (page 282). Even the peppery, bitter seeds can be eaten and are said to help get rid of intestinal worms. Papaya, particularly when unripe, is a wonderful digestive aid because of a powerful enzyme called papain, which helps break down proteins. The fruit is very soothing for the gut, helping to reduce inflammation and encouraging the elimination of gas and waste products. This is partly because of its rich fiber content, which also helps balance good bacteria in the gut and control cholesterol levels. The papain is also useful in helping calm inflammation elsewhere in the body, such as in the joints. As its color suggests, papaya is full of beta-carotene, as well as vitamin C.

papaya & shrimp salad

I FIRST MADE THIS WHEN I WAS LIVING IN BANGKOK, WHERE DELICIOUSLY FRESH
PAPAYAS WERE ABUNDANT AND INEXPENSIVE, BUT COTTAGE CHEESE WAS A RARITY!

2 ripe **papayas**
1 cup cottage cheese
8 oz cooked peeled shrimp
4 **scallions**, trimmed and
   finely sliced
juice of 1 **lime**
2 tsp tamari or soy sauce
2 heaped tsp **sesame seeds**

Cut the papayas in half and scoop out the seeds.
In a bowl, roughly mix together the cottage
cheese, shrimp, scallions, lime juice, and tamari,
using a fork. Pile the mixture into the papaya
cavities, sprinkle with the sesame seeds, and
eat immediately.

pan-grilled papaya with lime honey

HERE IS ANOTHER CONCOCTION INSPIRED BY MY DAYS IN BANGKOK, WHERE YOU COME ACROSS STREET-HAWKERS SELLING PEELED SLICES OF PAPAYA SPRINKLED WITH LIME JUICE—A SUBLIME FUSION. YOU WILL PROBABLY NEED TO COOK THE PAPAYA SLICES IN TWO OR THREE BATCHES.

*juice of 2 **limes***
*2 tsp **honey***
*1/2-inch piece fresh **ginger**, peeled and grated*
*2 **papayas**, peeled and sliced*

Preheat a ridged, castiron grill pan. In a bowl, mix together the lime juice, honey, and ginger. Swish the papaya slices around in the mixture, then lay them in the hot grill pan. Cook the papaya slices for about 2 minutes each side, brushing them with the marinade. Serve them hot, as they are or with plain yogurt.

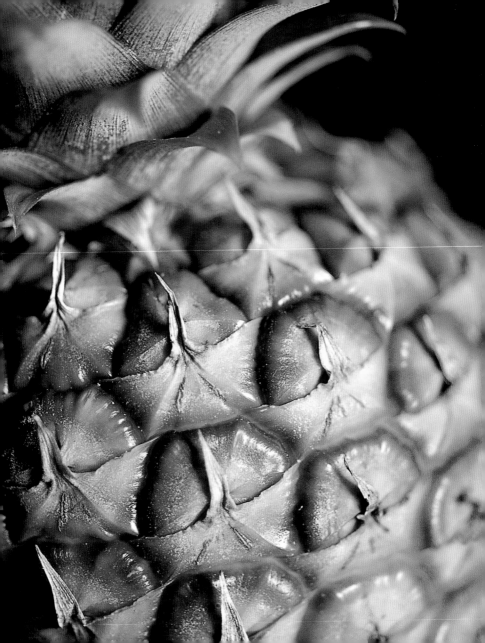

pineapple

Pineapples were so esteemed in 18th-century Europe that they were used as prestigious table decorations, and to this day, their sweet taste of the tropics is highly prized. A pineapple is actually a collection of flowers, each with its own "eye," fused around a central core. Fresh pineapple is rich in an enzyme called bromelain, which not only helps digestion but can also reduce inflammation. Eaten with a meal, pineapple helps the breakdown of proteins. It is so efficient at this that it is used as a meat tenderizer. For its anti-inflammatory effects, pineapple is best eaten between meals; this way it can help relieve the swelling linked to arthritis and sore throats, as well as injuries or operations. Bromelain appears to thin mucus, so it's useful for helping bronchitis, asthma, and sinus problems. It also helps reduce the stickiness of blood, and has been shown to relieve angina and thrombosis. Pineapple's high water content, combined with various acids it contains, gives it a diuretic action, which means it can be helpful for high blood pressure.

pineapple fish curry

LIGHT FISH AND TANGY PINEAPPLE CONTRAST WITH RICH COCONUT IN THIS
DELICIOUS CURRY. IF YOU CAN'T FIND KAFFIR LIME LEAVES, JUST LEAVE THEM OUT.

8 oz chunky **fish** fillet, such
as monkfish, skinned
2 tsp olive oil
1 medium **onion**, peeled
and finely diced
1-inch piece fresh **ginger**,
peeled and grated
1 lemongrass stalk, sliced
2 kaffir lime leaves, sliced
3 tbsp Thai red curry paste
$1/2$ fresh **pineapple**, peeled,
cored, and cubed
$2^{1}/_{2}$ cups **coconut** milk
12–15 **basil** leaves
6–8 cilantro sprigs, leaves
stripped off and torn

Cut the fish into bite-sized chunks and set aside.
Heat the olive oil in a large saucepan and cook the
onion with the ginger, lemongrass, and kaffir lime
leaves, stirring, until the onion is soft, 3–4 minutes.
Add the Thai curry paste and stir for a couple
of minutes.

Put the fish in the pan and toss gently for a
few minutes to lightly sear the pieces all over, then
add the pineapple. Pour in the coconut milk and
let cook gently for about 15 minutes.

Just before serving, stir in the basil and torn
cilantro leaves. Serve with brown rice.

baked prosciutto & endive rolls

THIS MAKES A GOOD FIRST COURSE. THE COMBINATION OF FLAVORS—BITTER, SWEET, AND SALTY—WORKS BRILLIANTLY.

4 heads of Belgian endive
16 **basil** leaves
½ small **pineapple**, peeled, cored, and chopped
freshly ground black pepper
8 slices of prosciutto or Serrano ham
1 tbsp balsamic vinegar
¼ cup freshly grated Parmesan cheese

Preheat the oven to 350°F. Slice the endive in half lengthwise and lay two basil leaves and three or four pieces of pineapple on each half. Grind a little black pepper over them and wrap each firmly in a slice of prosciutto.

Lay the rolls in a baking dish and pour in enough water to just cover the bottom of the dish. Cover with foil and bake for 20 minutes.

Remove the foil, sprinkle the balsamic vinegar over the rolls, and scatter the Parmesan over. Continue baking until the cheese has melted and the endive is soft, about 10 minutes longer.

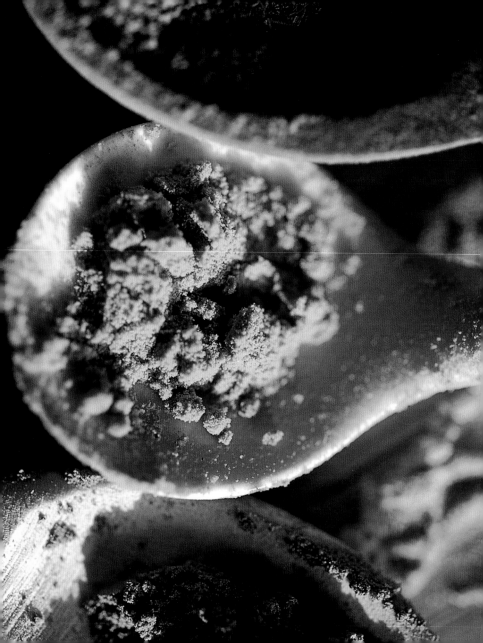

spices

Given their amazing aromas, tastes, and health benefits, it's no surprise that wars were fought over spices in past centuries. One of my favorite flavors ever is that of cardamom, which is wonderful in both sweet and savory dishes. Herbalists recommend it, as well as cinnamon, turmeric, and cloves, for their gut-soothing properties, which help expel wind, quell nausea, and calm gripey pains. Cinnamon is also renowned for its ability to relieve colds, arthritis, and high blood pressure. Turmeric, a root related to ginger, is often called "poor man's saffron" due to its color, but it is an outstanding spice in its own right. It contains curcumin, which has been widely researched for its abilities to help liver function; as a powerful anti-inflammatory, it is useful in cases of arthritis, Crohn's disease, and ulcerative colitis. Curcumin has even been shown to help protect against cancer. Cloves were an ancient remedy for toothache and, apart from pain relief, they are used to ease the symptoms of coughs and colds.

apple rice pudding

THIS MAY NOT BE LOADED WITH SUGAR AND CREAM LIKE A TRADITIONAL PUDDING, BUT TRY IT AND YOU'LL SEE HOW GOOD IT IS. FOR A RICE PUDDING IT'S RELATIVELY QUICK, BECAUSE YOU START OFF COOKING THE RICE ON THE STOVETOP—IN FACT, IT IS GREAT FOR USING UP LEFTOVER RICE.

$^3/_4$ cup **brown rice**
10 **cardamom** pods
1 **cinnamon** stick
$1^1/_2$ cups milk or **soymilk**
1 heaped tbsp sugar or
    alternative equivalent
    (see page 10)
1 heaped tbsp raisins
$^1/_2$ **apple**, peeled, cored,
    and grated
1 vanilla bean
1 tsp butter
blueberries or **strawberries**
    for serving

Cook the rice as instructed on the package, with the cardamom pods and cinnamon stick. In the meantime, preheat the oven to 350°F. Drain the rice, if necessary.

Heat the milk in a saucepan and stir in the rice, sugar, raisins, grated apple, vanilla bean, and butter. Tip the mixture into a small baking dish and stir well. Bake for 30 minutes.

Serve with fresh berries and, if you really want to splash out, some cream.

spicy masala tea

THIS BLEND OF DELICIOUS SPICES MAKES A WARMING, WINTER TEA. YOU COULD
ADD A LITTLE HONEY AS A SWEETENER, IF DESIRED.

½-inch piece fresh **ginger**,
   peeled and finely sliced
6 **cardamom** pods
1 **cinnamon** stick
5 **cloves**
2 cups water

Put all the ingredients in a large saucepan and
bring to a boil. Lower the heat and let simmer for
at least 10 minutes. Strain and serve.

NOTE You can leave the pan on the stovetop and
reheat the tea later when you fancy another cup, or
even keep it for a couple of days, replenishing the
water and perhaps adding a few extra spices. The
flavor of the cardamom in particular is more
pronounced the following day.

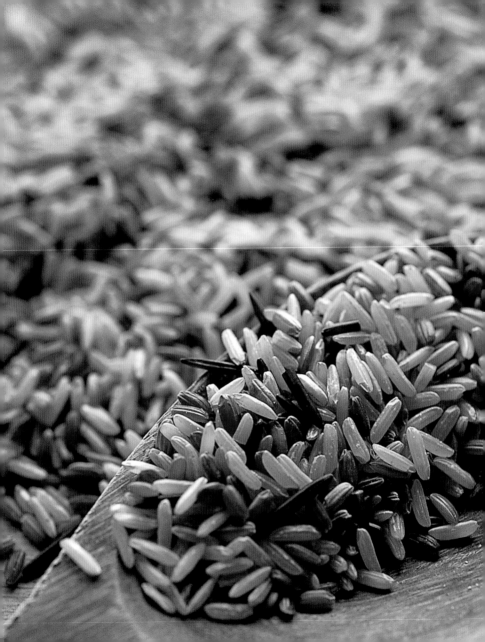

brown rice

Brown rice is slowly losing its reputation as worthy "hippy food," as more people appreciate its taste and texture, not to mention the nutrient value. It is simply the whole rice grain that has had only the outer hull removed. The process that transforms brown rice into white rice removes most of the vitamin stores, at least half of the minerals, all of the dietary fiber, and all of the essential fatty acids. Fiber is best known for encouraging healthy bowel movements; in keeping the elimination of wastes regular, you minimize your risk of problems such as diverticulitis and even colon cancer. Fiber also slows down the release of the starch as sugar into the bloodstream, making for a more satisfying meal and a steady release of energy. Rice is a naturally gluten-free starch, important for people who cannot digest gluten grains such as wheat and oats. Many people make the mistake of not cooking brown rice for long enough so it ends up *al dente* rather than slightly chewy.

mushroom risotto

THIS IS A REMARKABLY "CLEAN-FEELING" RISOTTO COMPARED WITH THE HEAVIER VERSIONS MADE WITH CREAM. IT'S GREAT AS A MAIN COURSE SERVED WITH A WONDERFOODS GREEN SALAD (PAGE 111). MISO IS A JAPANESE-STYLE SOYBEAN PASTE SOLD IN MOST HEALTHFOOD STORES AND MANY SUPERMARKETS.

3 tbsp miso (**soy** paste)
3³/₄ cups water
1¹/₄ cups white wine
1 heaped tbsp dried **seaweed**, such as arame
4 **shallots**, peeled and finely diced
2 **garlic** cloves, peeled and crushed
1 tbsp olive oil
7 oz shiitake **mushrooms**, sliced
¹/₂-inch piece fresh **ginger**, peeled and finely sliced
1 fresh, hot red chile, seeded and sliced
1¹/₄ cups **brown rice**
1 heaped tbsp torn cilantro leaves

In one saucepan, mix the miso with the water and wine, add the seaweed, and bring to a simmer.

In another pan, soften the shallots and garlic in the olive oil until translucent, then add the mushrooms, ginger, and chile. Stir for a few minutes before adding the rice.

Turn up the heat under the miso mixture to bring it to a boil, then add it to the rice. Stir and cover with the lid. Turn down to the lowest setting and let cook gently for 40 minutes.

To serve, pile the risotto on plates and top with a sprinkling of cilantro leaves.

scented savory rice

THIS IS A WONDERFULLY AROMATIC WAY OF COOKING RICE, ESPECIALLY TO
ACCOMPANY A DISH SUCH AS MOROCCAN LAMB (PAGE 194).

1¹/₄ cups **brown rice**
3 cups water
6 **cardamom** pods
4 **cloves**
¹/₂ **cinnamon** stick
¹/₂ tsp ground **turmeric**

Put all the ingredients in a large saucepan and
bring to a boil. Cover with a lid and turn the heat
down to a simmer. Cook until the rice is soft and
chewy rather than *al dente*; this should take about
40 minutes. (I usually cheat and use an electric
rice cooker, which gets the water evaporation right
every time.)

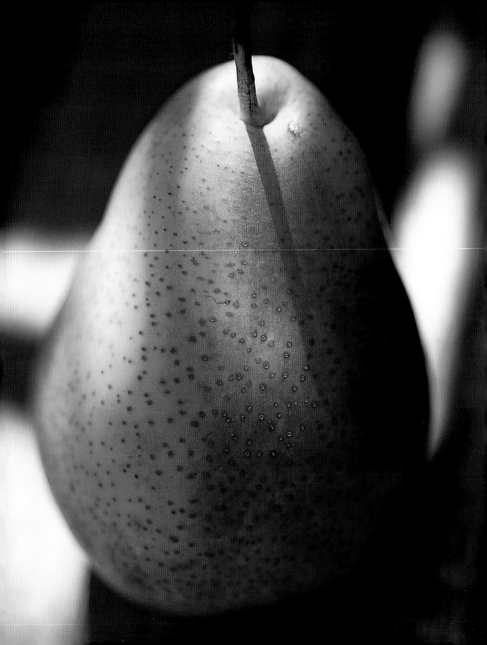

pear

When you bite into a ripe pear and the juice dribbles down your chin, you can see why Homer referred to this fruit as a "gift of the gods." Pears have much in common with their distant relative, the apple: many shapes, sizes, hues, and health benefits. Pears are higher in the soluble fiber pectin than apples, which make them very cleansing and soothing for the whole digestive tract. Not only does pectin help keep the bowels moving well, it also binds to waste products and cancer-causing substances in the colon. When ripe, pears are very easy to break down, which makes them gentle on the digestion and a good source of energy that, combined with the fiber, releases only gradually. Pears are generally considered one of the foods least likely to trigger an allergic reaction, so they are an ideal fruit to introduce to babies being weaned and anyone with a sensitive system. Unlike many fruits, pears are best ripened after picking, so they turn buttery and don't develop a grainy texture.

pear & feta salad

MY PREFERRED VARIETY OF PEAR IS BARTLETT, BUT YOU CAN USE ANY TYPE YOU
LIKE. AND YOU CAN REPLACE THE FETA WITH GOAT CHEESE OR EVEN A GOOD
BLUE CHEESE.

*2 ripe but firm **pears***
5 oz feta cheese
*5 oz **spinach**, washed*
4 oz arugula, washed
*¹/₂ cup **walnut** halves*
2 tsp balsamic vinegar
*1 tbsp **walnut** oil*

Quarter the pears lengthwise, remove the cores, and then cut into eighths. Cut the feta cheese into eight slices.

Toss the spinach, arugula, and walnuts with the balsamic vinegar and walnut oil, and pile on four plates. Arrange the pear and feta slices on top and serve.

morning zing juice

THE TASTE AND TEXTURE OF MELON JUICE SOMEHOW CONJURE UP THE SENSATION OF CREAMINESS, ALL OFFSET BY THE SHARP GINGER AND SWEET MINT.

*3 ripe but firm **pears***
*1 thick slice of **melon**,
    peeled and seeded*
*¹/₂-inch piece fresh **ginger**,
    peeled*
small bunch of mint

Chop the pears and melon into pieces small enough to fit through the opening of your juicer. Push all the ingredients through, one by one, and drink the juice right away. Well, after you've washed up the juicer perhaps!

NOTE If you don't have a juicer, you can make a smoothie using a blender, but you will need to use slightly over-ripe pears. Peel, core, and chop the pears; chop the melon; and grate the ginger. Whiz in a blender with the mint, then thin with a little water, if necessary.

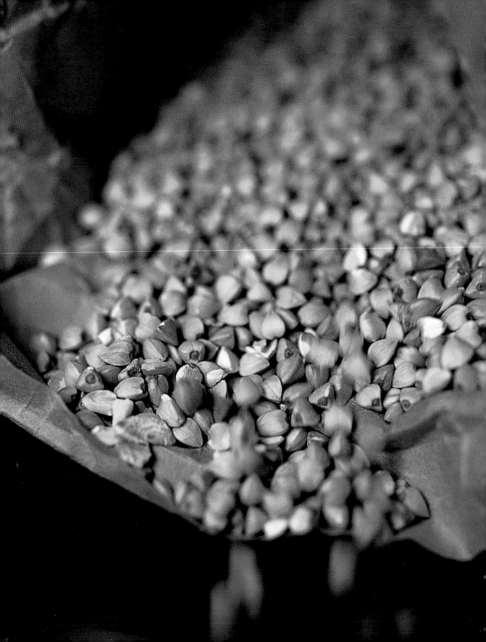

buckwheat

Buckwheat was introduced into Europe by the Crusaders and later the Turks, which is how it got its original name, "Saracen wheat." Contrary to the name, buckwheat isn't a grain, but a fruit seed related to rhubarb. This makes it a good alternative for anyone avoiding the gluten grains (wheat, oats, rye, and barley), including people who find gluten triggers digestive problems or depression. Buckwheat contains fiber and all eight essential amino acids, so, for a grainlike food, it is a good source of protein. Although it's not particularly high in the amino acid tryptophan, the carb content means there's more chance of the tryptophan being converted to serotonin, which boosts moods. The rich magnesium in buckwheat is useful for relaxing the nervous system and muscles—including those in the bowel, which can alleviate constipation. Buckwheat is notably rich in an antioxidant called rutin, which helps to strengthen blood capillaries and prevent the platelets in the blood from clotting together.

buckwheat crêpes

WE USUALLY HAVE THESE WITH BLUEBERRIES AND PLAIN YOGURT, OR SCRAMBLED EGGS AND SPINACH, ON A SUNDAY MORNING.

*1 cup **buckwheat** flour*
pinch of salt
*1 **egg***
*²/₃ cup milk or **soymilk***
²/₃ cup water
splash of olive oil

Put the flour and salt in a mixing bowl, make a well in the middle, and add the egg. Mix the milk and water together. Beat the egg into the flour, then gradually add the liquid, plus a splash of olive oil, to make a smooth batter. Ideally, let the batter stand for at least 1 hour.

When you're ready to cook the crêpes, lightly oil a frying pan and heat it well. Pour in about 1 tbsp batter and tilt the pan around to spread the batter to the edge. Cook until the crêpe is golden underneath, 1–2 minutes, then flip it over and cook the other side for a minute or so. Remove the crêpes and stack on a warm plate, separating them with wax paper; keep warm. Repeat with the rest of the batter.

Serve the crêpes with your choice of topping, sweet or savory.

soba noodles & salmon

SOBA ARE JAPANESE NOODLES MADE WITH BUCKWHEAT FLOUR. THEY HAVE A VERY DISTINCT FLAVOR.

10 oz dried soba
    (**buckwheat**) noodles
grated zest of 1 **lime**
juice of 2 **limes**
1 small, fresh, hot chile,
    seeded and sliced
1 heaped tbsp brown sugar
1 tsp ground coriander
1 tbsp tamari or soy sauce
4 small **salmon** fillets
splash of olive oil
4 **shallots**, peeled and
    finely diced
1 tbsp toasted **sesame** oil
2 heaped tbsp chopped
    cilantro leaves

Cook the soba noodles in a pan of boiling water until *al dente*, 6–8 minutes. Drain, rinse in cold water, and drain again well.

In a bowl, mix together the lime zest and juice, chile, sugar, ground coriander, and tamari. Add the salmon fillets and turn to coat them in the mixture; set aside.

Heat a wok, add a splash of olive oil, and soften the shallots until translucent. Add the salmon fillets along with the marinade and cook until done to your taste, 2–3 minutes each side— you could just sear them briefly. Remove the fish and set aside.

Add the noodles to the wok along with the sesame oil and toss to heat them through. Divide the noodles among four plates, lay a piece of salmon on each pile, and scatter the cilantro over.

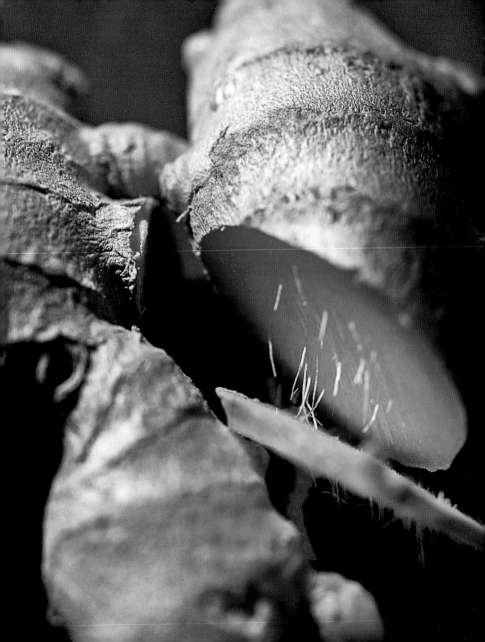

ginger

Ginger has been used for centuries as a medicinal and spiritual cleanser. In Ayurvedic and traditional Chinese medicine, it occurs in half of all prescriptions. The versatility of this hot, refreshing, juicy root makes it a good addition to both sweet and savory dishes, as well as to a medicine cabinet. Ginger's primary health uses are in calming the gut—it not only helps to quell nausea, but also to soothe gripes, diarrhea, and wind. Studies have suggested that it also has a role in preventing motion sickness and vomiting in pregnancy, as well as the ability to help ulcers heal. Several natural chemicals in ginger, including gingerols, inhibit inflammatory substances in the body, making it particularly useful for anyone with arthritis, asthma, or other conditions involving inflammation. On the cardiovascular front, ginger reduces the stickiness of blood, tones the heart, and reduces cholesterol levels. In addition to treating digestive upsets and respiratory tract infections, Western herbalists also recommend ginger as a stimulant that warms the body and boosts circulation.

baked gingered fish

YOU CAN USE ANY WHITE FISH FOR THIS DISH, BUT MY FAVORITE IS THE
DELICIOUS, RICH, ANTARCTIC ICEFISH.

*4 white **fish** steaks*
¹⁄₄ cup water
FOR THE MARINADE
*1-inch piece fresh **ginger**,*
  peeled and grated
*2 **garlic** cloves, peeled*
  and crushed
grated zest and juice of
  *1 **lime***
2 tsp tamari or soy sauce
1 fresh, hot red chile, seeded
  and sliced

Combine all the ingredients for the marinade in a
shallow baking dish. Add the fish steaks and turn
to coat them in the mixture. Ideally, set aside to
marinate for 2 or 3 hours, but if you don't have the
time, you'll find the dish still tastes great.

Preheat the oven to 400°F. Add the water to the
marinade in the dish and stir it in well. Bake until
the fish steaks are cooked through, 15–20 minutes.
Icefish usually takes a little longer than most other
white fish, because the texture is quite dense.

Eat with stir-fried vegetables and a little brown
rice or Herby sweet oven fries (page 198).

roasted pears with lime & ginger

THIS EASY-TO-PREPARE DESSERT CAN BE KEPT IN THE REFRIGERATOR FOR A COUPLE OF DAYS—YOU MIGHT EVEN BE TEMPTED TO HAVE SOME FOR BREAKFAST. THE PEARS CAN BE CUT UP AND COOKED IN THE PAN WITH THE SYRUP, IF PREFERRED, TO MAKE A SORT OF COMPOTE.

1 cup water
1-inch piece fresh **ginger**,
    peeled and finely sliced
1 tbsp **honey**
grated zest and juice of
    1 **lime**
1/2 cup white wine
4 ripe but firm **pears**
FOR SERVING
6 heaped tbsp plain **yogurt**
3/4 tsp ground **cinnamon**
1/2 tsp vanilla extract
4 mint leaves (optional)

Preheat the oven to 350°F. Put the water, ginger, honey, and lime juice and zest in a saucepan. Bring to a boil, then add the wine. Let simmer for 10 minutes.

Meanwhile, quarter and core the pears and lay them in a baking dish. Pour the ginger and lime mixture over the pears and bake them for about 30 minutes.

Mix the yogurt with the cinnamon and vanilla extract. When the pears are tender, place two halves on each plate. Top with a dollop of the flavored yogurt and, if you're feeling fancy, finish with a mint leaf.

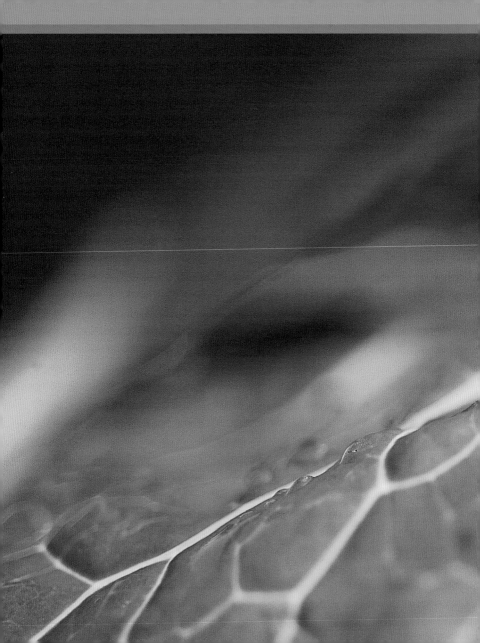

detox

Detoxing has become something of a buzz word in the last few years and countless books have been published on detox programs. This is not what this section of Wonderfoods is about! The foods here are ones that contain nutrients which enhance the body's natural, ongoing, normal detoxification processes. It's easy to forget, with the books and magazine articles on detoxing, that it is something our bodies do permanently—every hour of every day. The wonderfoods here can help to optimize that process.

Although all cells do their own housework throughout the body, the liver is the main organ of detoxification. It is best known for processing challenging substances like alcohol, but this vital organ has many roles. Its other important tasks include storing glucose and helping balance blood levels of this crucial fuel, storing other nutrients, breaking down fats, making cholesterol, forming proteins, and producing bile salts to help with digestion.

So making sure the liver is in good shape is vital for health. If this key organ is being overwhelmed, you're likely to feel tired, sluggish, and achey and have poor digestion or bad skin. All the wonderfoods in this section are rich in antioxidant nutrients, which the liver needs in high doses. From humble vitamin C to the glucosinolates in broccoli and kale, a spectrum of antioxidants keeps the liver ticking over well. Another nutrient required for detoxification in the liver is sulfur. It is generally recognized that a common reason for feeling run down and sluggish is exceeding your body's capacity to detoxify what you put in it.

To keep your detox processes working efficiently you need to load up on the foods that are good for your liver, such as the wonderfoods in this section, and minimize your intake of foods and other substances that tax it. So cutting back on alcohol, caffeine, fatty foods, salty foods, processed sugars, and food additives lessens the burden on your body's detox capacity. Even before "detox diet" became trendy, many cultures had for hundreds of years valued periods of abstention from such substances for both spiritual and health reasons, and we would do well to follow suit.

Many people find that lightening the load on their liver and boosting it with selected foods such as the detox wonderfoods makes them feel energized, alert, and clearer in both their mind and body.

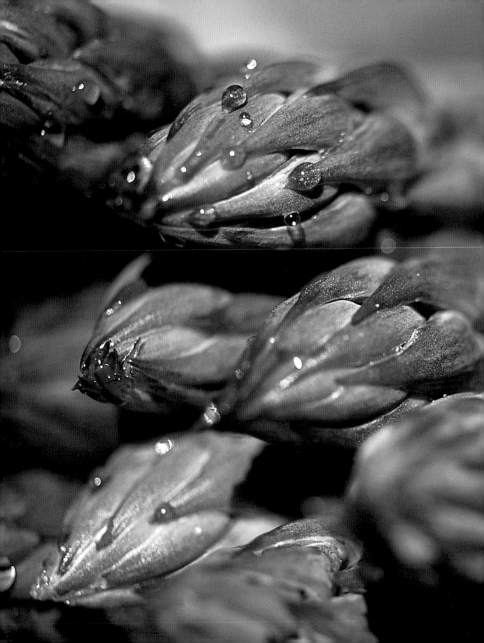

asparagus

Asparagus was cultivated in all corners of the Roman empire and was known as "sparrowgrass" in Britain in the 18th century. Not only is it still a delicacy, this vegetable is loaded with goodness. In one serving, you get about a third of your daily need for folic acid, which is not only crucial for the proper development of a baby but also good heart health. Asparagus also contains an amino acid called asparagine. This, along with its high potassium content and low sodium, makes asparagus a diuretic and cleanser, useful for processing proteins and flushing out the kidneys. Diuretics not only help reduce blood pressure, but also water retention in the legs and premenstrually. Asparagus is a source of the flavonoid rutin, which has an affinity for healthy blood capillaries, helping prevent them from rupturing, such as in hemorrhoids. Because of its phallic shape, asparagus was considered to be an aphrodisiac, but, unfortunately, it doesn't actually seem to have any chemical properties that would make that true.

pan-grilled asparagus with serrano ham

THE FINER THE ASPARAGUS SPEARS, THE MORE TENDER AND SWEET THEY ARE. IF YOU CAN GET HOLD OF IT, WHITE ASPARAGUS MAKES THIS DISH A REAL DELICACY.

splash of olive oil
1 tbsp balsamic vinegar
*16–20 **asparagus** spears*
8 slices of Serrano ham
  (or prosciutto)

Heat a splash of olive oil and the balsamic vinegar in a well-seasoned, ridged, castiron grill pan or nonstick frying pan. When it's hot, add the asparagus spears and cook until lightly charred on one side. Turn and cook them on the other side until they are just limp. Arrange the asparagus on plates with the slices of Serrano ham and serve.

asparagus-chicken stir-fry

BECAUSE ASPARAGUS AND CHICKEN BOTH HAVE QUITE DELICATE FLAVORS, NEITHER CROWDS OUT THE OTHER IN THIS LIGHT MEAL.

a little toasted sesame oil
*2 **shallots**, peeled and finely diced*
*1 **garlic** clove, peeled and crushed*
3/4 tsp Chinese five spice powder
*2 large, boneless **chicken** breast halves, skinned and sliced*
*12 thin **asparagus** spears, trimmed and sliced*
2 tbsp water
2 tsp tamari or soy sauce
*2 heaped tsp **sesame seeds***

Heat a wok and add a little sesame oil, then add the shallots and garlic with the five spice powder and sauté until softened. Add the chicken slices and toss over the heat for a few minutes until the chicken is nearly cooked through.

Add the asparagus, water, and tamari, and toss well, then cover and cook for a couple of minutes until the asparagus and chicken are cooked.

Serve the stir-fry sprinkled with sesame seeds, on a bed of rice noodles.

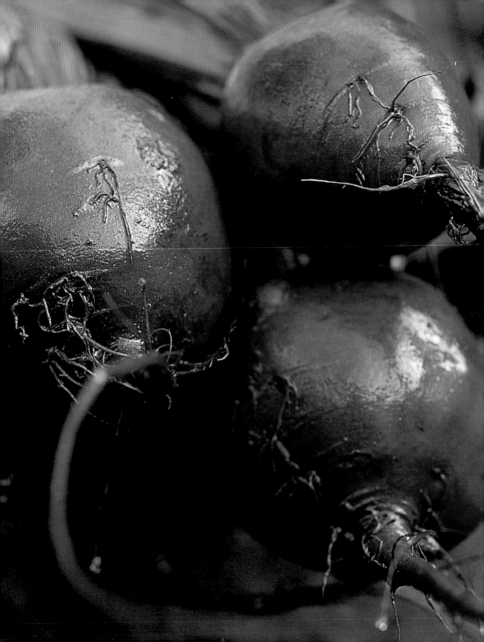

beets

Stunningly colored beets are loaded with nutrients and, as their hues suggest, are considered very purifying for the blood. They have been used over the centuries as folk remedies for anemia, menstrual problems, and kidney disorders, and now modern science is revealing their wonders. One constituent of this root vegetable that contributes to the deep red color is betacyanin. This and other powerful antioxidants in beets have been shown to enhance detoxing processes in the liver and even help protect against cancer of the skin, lungs, and colon. Studies have indicated that beet extracts increase the activity of the body's natural antioxidant enzymes in the liver, such as glutathione peroxidase. Beets have also been shown to help lower cholesterol and increase the ratio of the HDL "good cholesterol" to the LDL "bad" type. In addition to the roots, beet tops (or leaves) are highly nutritious—loaded with iron and beta-carotene. Beets are most commonly eaten boiled, but are also wonderful roasted, and eaten raw—particularly if they are grated.

marinated red onion & beet salad

IF YOU'RE NOT USED TO HAVING RAW BEETS, THIS IS A GOOD RECIPE TO START
WITH. YOU CAN REPLACE THE FETA WITH A GOOD GOAT CHEESE, IF PREFERRED.

2 medium **beets**, peeled
   and grated
½ red **onion**, peeled and
   very finely sliced
juice of 1½ **lemons**
1 tbsp olive oil
1 heaped tbsp chopped
   parsley
fine sea salt
2 handfuls of **watercress**,
   trimmed
5 oz feta cheese, crumbled

In a bowl, toss the grated beets and slivers of
red onion with the lemon juice. Let marinate,
ideally overnight.

Just before serving, mix in the olive oil and
chopped parsley and season with a little sea salt.

Arrange the watercress on plates, spoon on the
beet mixture, and top with crumbled feta. Serve
with hot rye bread.

roasted beet soup

THIS VIVID SOUP IS EQUALLY GOOD HOT OR COLD. A SWIRL OF PLAIN YOGURT IS THE PERFECT CONTRAST.

2¼ lb **beets**, peeled and
    chopped
1 large **onion**, cut into
    8 wedges (unpeeled)
2 heaped tsp caraway seeds
4–6 **thyme** sprigs
freshly ground black pepper
olive oil for drizzling
1 cup chicken or vegetable
    stock
juice of ½ **lemon**
FOR SERVING
plain **yogurt**
2 heaped tbsp chopped
    parsley

Preheat the oven to 350°F. Put the beets and onion pieces in a roasting pan with the caraway seeds and thyme. Season with pepper, drizzle with olive oil, and toss well. Roast until the beets feel tender when pierced with a skewer, 30–40 minutes.

Remove the papery skin from the onion, then tip the contents of the pan into a large saucepan. Add the stock and lemon juice and heat gently to a simmer. Remove from the heat and whiz to a smooth consistency using an immersion blender (or use a free-standing blender, then reheat gently to serve hot).

As you serve the soup, top each portion with a spoonful of yogurt and swirl decoratively. Sprinkle with the chopped parsley.

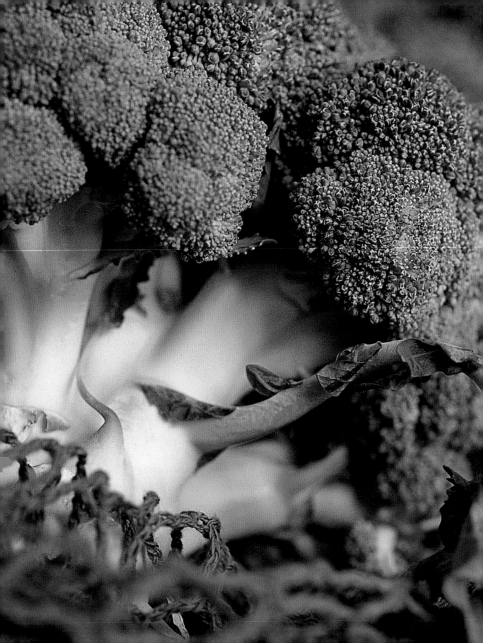

broccoli & kale

Broccoli and kale are just two members of the cruciferous family, so called because of the crosslike structure of their stems. Brussels sprouts, cabbage, cauliflower and broccoli rabe are cousins. Kale and broccoli in particular are two of the most power-packed veggies! Broccoli is rich in vitamin C and kale is one of the highest antioxidant foods there is. Both are excellent sources of fiber, which helps keep the bowel working efficiently and feeds good bacteria there. Broccoli and kale are also rich sources of glucosinolates, which have powerful actions in the detoxification processes in the liver. Of these, sulforaphane, sinigrin, and indole-3-carbinol (I3C), have been found to be powerful anti-cancer substances. I3C is involved in processing estrogen, helping balance menstrual cycles, and potentially protecting against breast cancer. Both—but kale in particular—are loaded with beta-carotene and its relatives, lutein and zeaxanthin. These chemicals are good for immunity, but especially for protecting the eye against sunlight damage and age-related macular degeneration.

broccoli & sweet potato salad

THIS WONDERFUL COMBINATION FIRST PASSED MY LIPS IN A CAFE IN AUCKLAND, NEW ZEALAND, AND IT'S BEEN A FIRM LUNCH FAVORITE IN OUR HOUSE EVER SINCE.

2 **sweet potatoes**, scrubbed and cut into ½-inch disks
1 red **bell pepper**, cored, seeded, and sliced
3–4 **thyme** sprigs
olive oil for drizzling
1 head of **broccoli**, cut into florets
5 oz feta cheese, cubed
1 heaped tbsp **sunflower seeds**
1 tbsp cider vinegar
freshly ground black pepper

Preheat the oven to 350°F. Put the sweet potatoes, red pepper, and thyme sprigs in a roasting pan and drizzle with some olive oil. Toss well, then roast until the sweet potatoes are tender, about 30 minutes. Set aside to cool.

Meanwhile, plunge the broccoli florets into a pan of boiling water and blanch for no more than a minute. Drain and refresh in cold water, then drain thoroughly.

When all the vegetables are cool, toss them in a bowl with the feta, sunflower seeds, cider vinegar, pepper to taste, and a little more olive oil. Serve at once.

green spice stir-fry

IF I'M COOKING A FISH OR MEAT CURRY, I FIND THIS IS A GOOD, LIGHT DISH TO
SERVE ALONGSIDE, RATHER THAN MAKING ANOTHER SAUCY CURRY.

1 heaped tsp cumin seeds
1 tbsp olive oil
1 **garlic** clove, peeled and
    crushed
1 small, fresh, hot chile,
    seeded and sliced
1 head of **broccoli**, cut into
    florets
8–10 **kale** leaves, torn off
    the stems
2 tbsp water

Toast the cumin seeds in a dry wok over moderate
heat until they are lightly browned and giving off a
lovely aroma. Add the olive oil, garlic, and chile,
and stir for a minute or two, then add the broccoli,
kale, and water. Stir over the heat for a few minutes
until the kale leaves are wilted and the broccoli is
cooked through but still slightly crunchy.

Serve at once, with brown rice and Moroccan
lamb (page 194) or Pineapple fish curry (page 58).

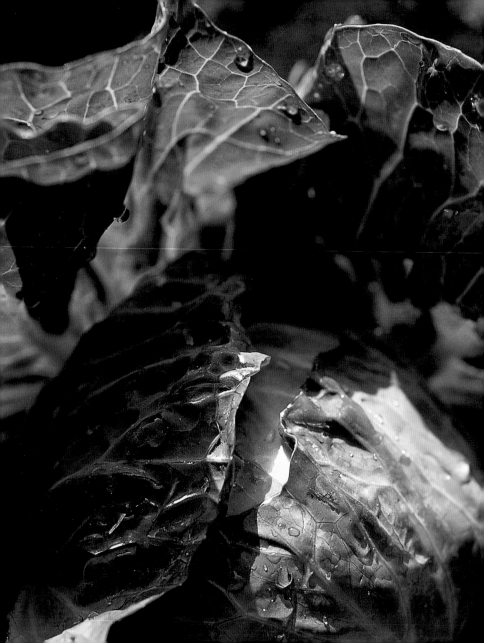

cabbage

The humble, common cabbage may not be the classiest of vegetables, but it is one of the richest, healthwise. Even ancient Egyptians knew how good it was for the liver—apparently they ate loads in advance of drinking binges! Like its relatives broccoli and kale, cabbage contains a range of powerful, sulfurous substances that protect the liver, boost its detox capacity, aid the processing of hormones, and can even help protect against certain cancers. Sulfur, sometimes referred to as the "beauty mineral," is also needed for healthy skin, hair, and nails. Cabbage juice, although hardly a gastronomic delight, is a traditional remedy for peptic ulcers. In addition to their high fiber content, cabbages are packed with nutrients such as vitamin C, folic acid, calcium, potassium, and many more. Cabbage that is overcooked and soggy is unpalatable, but lightly blanched or stir-fried, or even shredded raw in salads, it's delicious. Red cabbage has even more goodness than white or green, plus a striking touch of color.

keralan cabbage

WHILE BEING PUNTED ALONG THE TRANQUIL BACKWATERS OF KERALA IN SOUTHERN INDIA, I FEASTED ON LOCAL DISHES PREPARED BY THOMAS THE CHEF, INCLUDING THIS ONE. YOU CAN BUY CURRY LEAVES, FRESH OR DRIED, FROM ASIAN MARKETS.

1 tbsp **coconut** oil (or olive oil)
1 heaped tsp mustard seeds
1 heaped tbsp curry leaves
1 fresh, hot green chile, seeded and finely sliced
1 heaped tsp cumin seeds
3/4 tsp ground **turmeric**
1/2-inch piece fresh **ginger**, peeled and grated
2 heaped tbsp grated **coconut** (ideally fresh, otherwise use dried)
1 **onion**, peeled and very finely diced
1/3 head of **cabbage**, very finely shredded

Heat a wok and add the oil (ideally coconut). Throw in the mustard seeds, curry leaves, chile, cumin seeds, turmeric, and ginger, and stir for a minute or two. Add the coconut and onion and cook, stirring, for 3–4 minutes.

Add the cabbage to the spice mixture and stir and toss for about 5 minutes. Serve immediately, with spicy grilled fish and rice.

salmon rolls

VIETNAMESE SPRING ROLLS AND CHINESE DUCK PANCAKES WERE THE INSPIRATION FOR THESE! OTHER THAN TASTING FANTASTIC, THEY ARE A FUN WAY TO SHARE FOOD AROUND A TABLE WITH FRIENDS.

4 small **salmon** fillets

12 large Savoy **cabbage** leaves (at least)

½ English **cucumber**, cut into strips

4–6 **scallions**, trimmed and finely shredded lengthwise

large handful of **bean sprouts**

8–10 tbsp tamari or soy sauce

1-inch piece fresh **ginger**, peeled and grated

3 tbsp toasted **sesame** oil

Steam or poach the salmon until just tender. Roughly break it up with a fork, then tip it into a serving bowl and let cool.

Bring a large saucepan of water to a boil and blanch the cabbage leaves until pliable, about 2 minutes. Drain and refresh under cold water, then drain well and place on a serving plate.

Arrange the cucumber, scallions, and bean sprouts on another serving plate. Mix the tamari, grated ginger, and sesame oil in two small serving bowls or individual dipping bowls.

Put all the serving dishes on the table and let guests help themselves. To eat, you simply roll some salmon and vegetables in a cabbage leaf and dip it into the sauce.

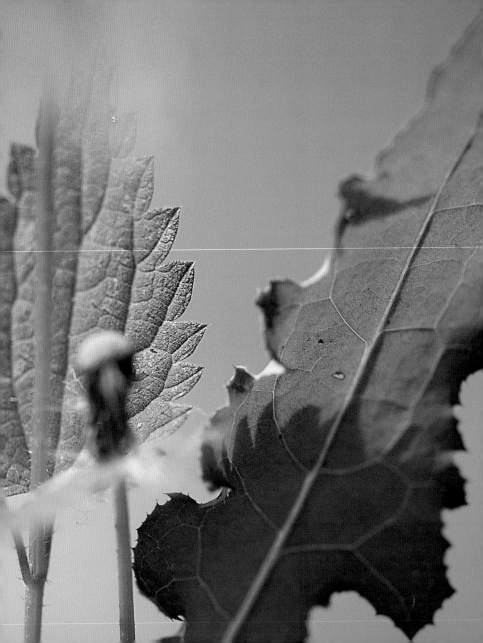

dandelion &
nettles

If you're a gardener you may see these as pernicious weeds and slay them at all costs. Before you do, pick the leaves and make the most of their outstanding properties. Spring is the best time to harvest dandelion, when the leaves are at their most tender and sweet—eat them raw in salads or cooked, like spinach. The roots, too, are good, eaten raw or stir-fried. Dandelion is considered by herbalists to be one of the best liver tonics: It helps the actual liver detoxification and also the flow of bile to and from the gall bladder. The bitterness of the leaves stimulates digestion, especially of fats, and this, along with their soluble fiber, encourages bowel movements. Dandelion is also useful for combatting water retention. As for stinging nettles, don gloves to pick the young shoots at the top of the stems and cook them like spinach. The cooking process destroys the poison that makes them sting and you are left with flavorful greens that have been used for centuries to treat water retention and kidney disorders, and to stimulate the liver and digestion.

warm dandelion & sunchoke salad

ARGAN OIL FROM MOROCCO IS A WONDERFUL NUTTY OIL, RICH IN OMEGA-6 FATS. YOU CAN BUY IT FROM MOST HEALTHFOOD STORES AND WHOLEFOOD MARKETS.

8 **Jerusalem artichokes**, well scrubbed
juice of ½ **lemon**, plus a squeeze
1 heaped tbsp **pumpkin seeds**
handful of tender **dandelion** leaves
2 **scallions**, trimmed and sliced
1 heaped tbsp chopped **parsley**
1 tbsp argan oil
pinch of fine sea salt
freshly ground black pepper
5 oz goat cheese, crumbled

Boil the Jerusalem artichokes (sunchokes) in water to cover, with the juice of ½ lemon added, until they feel tender when pierced with a skewer, about 15 minutes. Drain and let cool.

Meanwhile, lightly toast the pumpkin seeds in a dry frying pan.

When the Jerusalem artichokes are cooked and cool, cut them into disks and combine with the dandelion leaves, pumpkin seeds, scallions, and parsley. Drizzle with the argan oil and a squeeze of lemon juice, and season with salt and pepper. Toss to mix and serve topped with the crumbled goat cheese.

mackerel with nettles

THIS "EXOTIC" RECIPE COMES FROM DORSET, ENGLAND, WHERE MY FRIEND JAMES VERNER FIRST ENCOURAGED ME TO TRY EATING NETTLES. IF YOU CANNOT STEAM THE NETTLES AS THE RECIPE SUGGESTS, RINSE THEM IN WATER AND COOK THEM IN A DRY SAUCEPAN AS YOU WOULD SPINACH. DRINK THE REMAINING LIQUID, WHICH IS VERY CLEANSING.

5 fresh, hot red chiles
1 **garlic** clove, peeled
handful of **sage, thyme,**
    and **parsley** leaves
2 tbsp olive oil
4 **mackerel**, cleaned,
    heads on
25 stinging **nettle** tips
dash of balsamic vinegar
4 **lemon** slices

Using a mortar and pestle, pound 1 halved and seeded chile with the garlic, herbs, and about 1 tbsp olive oil. Stuff the mixture into the fish cavities and secure the opening with wooden toothpicks. Preheat the broiler.

Steam the nettles until they lose their sting, about 5 minutes.

Meanwhile, cook the mackerel under the hot broiler for 3–4 minutes each side.

Toss the nettles in 1 tbsp olive oil and a dash of balsamic vinegar, then spread them out on plates. Lay a mackerel on each bed of nettles and garnish with a twist of lemon and a whole chile.

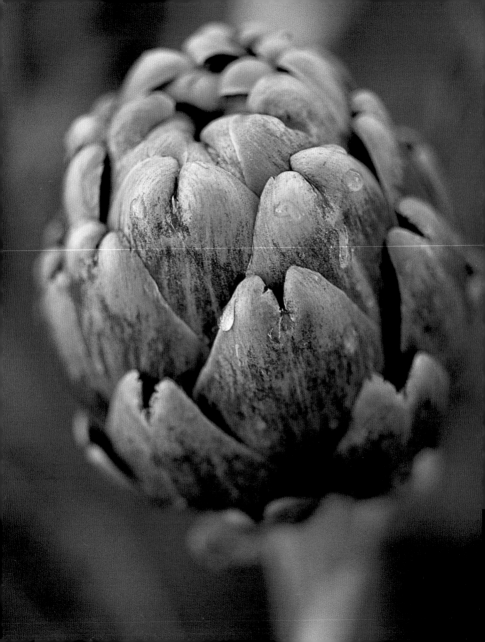

globe artichoke

Surprisingly, perhaps, this vegetable is a member of the thistle family. Medicinally, it is best known for supporting the liver and gall bladder, i.e. it is useful in boosting detoxification and digestion. This is particularly due to natural chemicals it contains, such as cynarin. Recent studies have even shown that extracts of artichoke can help relieve the symptoms of irritable bowel syndrome, such as nausea, pain, constipation, and wind. It also has antifungal properties. Herbalists recommend globe artichoke for its diuretic properties—helping relieve water retention and high blood pressure. Another bonus for the cardiovascular system is that globe artichoke has been shown to reduce levels of LDL, the so-called "bad cholesterol." Antioxidant flavonoids from the artichoke, such as luteolin, help to prevent LDL oxidation, which may reduce the risk of atherosclerosis, or thickening and hardening of the arteries. When you buy globe artichokes, it is the unopened flowerheads of the plant that are eaten—choose ones that feel heavy for their size.

stuffed artichokes

"POGGI POGGI" IS THE RIDICULOUS NAME IN OUR FAMILY (COINED BY MY COUSIN LIZZIE) FOR TRADITIONAL MALTESE STUFFED ARTICHOKES, AS PREPARED BY OUR GRANDMOTHER AND NOW BY MY AUNTIE MARLENE. THE PROPER MALTESE NAME IS *QAQOCC MIMLI*, WHERE THE "Q" HAS A GLOTTAL STOP SOUND.

4 large **globe artichokes**, trimmed
FOR THE STUFFING
6 slices of brown bread, toasted and crumbed
6 **garlic** cloves, peeled and crushed
4 anchovy fillets, chopped and mashed
large handful of flat-leaf **parsley**, finely chopped
1 heaped tbsp chopped **oregano**
3 tbsp olive oil
freshly ground black pepper
FOR SERVING
olive oil
squeeze of **lemon** juice

Mix all the stuffing ingredients together in a bowl. Take each artichoke and slam its top on the kitchen counter to open up the leaves. Push generous amounts of stuffing down in between the leaves.

Stand the artichokes in a large saucepan and add enough water to come 1 inch up their sides. Cover and steam until they are tender, about 40 minutes.

Serve each artichoke on a plate with a side dish of olive oil flavored with a little lemon juice in which to dip each leaf base as it is pulled. Scrape the flesh and accompanying stuffing off each leaf with your teeth before discarding the rough, hairy choke and enjoying the tender heart.

artichoke heart pizzas

THESE WONDERFUL APPETIZERS COULD BE MADE IN BULK TO SERVE AS CANAPÉS.
AS YOU'LL SEE, THE "PIZZA" BASE IS ACTUALLY AN ARTICHOKE HEART. YOU CAN
LEAVE OUT THE ANCHOVIES FOR A VEGETARIAN VERSION.

4 **shallots**, peeled and
 finely diced
1 **garlic** clove, peeled
 and crushed
a little olive oil
8 canned **artichoke** hearts
 (or from a jar), drained
1 heaped tsp chopped
 parsley
2 **tomatoes**, sliced
8 **basil** leaves
4 anchovies, cut in half
¹/₄ cup freshly grated
 Parmesan cheese
8 black olives, pitted
freshly ground black pepper
arugula leaves for serving

Preheat the oven to 350°F. In a small frying pan,
soften the shallots and garlic in a little olive oil
until translucent.

Lay the artichoke hearts in a baking pan and
spread a little of the cooked shallot mixture on
each, then sprinkle with the parsley. Layer the
tomato slices, basil leaves, anchovies, and grated
Parmesan on top. Add an olive to each, season
with pepper, and bake for 15–20 minutes.

Serve on a bed of arugula leaves.

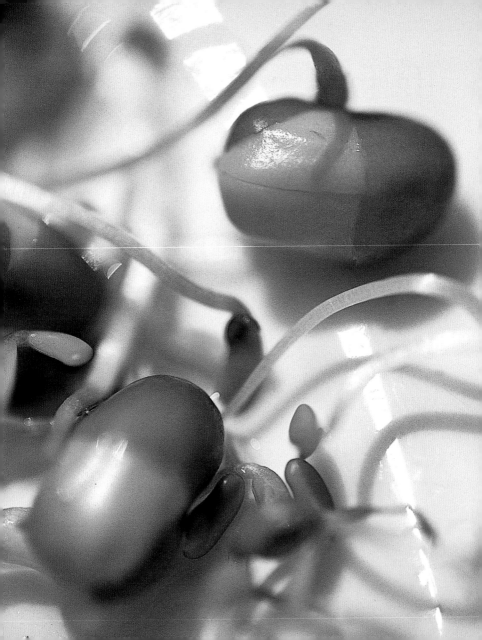

alfalfa & mung sprouts

Grow your own sprouts from dormant seeds and you can benefit from the concentrated nutrients they offer as they spring to life and become edible. Sprouts contain phytonutrients, similar, yet more condensed than those in the fully grown plant. For example, scientists estimate broccoli sprouts contain at least ten times the antioxidant power of mature broccoli. During sprouting, the activity of enzymes increases dramatically, converting the starch into simple sugars, protein into amino acids, and fats into fatty acids. These processes in effect pre-digest the seed, making it much easier for us to break it down and absorb the nutrients. Whatever the content of the sprouts (and they will, of course, differ from one to the other), the key is freshness. If you let sprouts develop leaves and expose them to sunshine so they turn green, you'll have a fresh source of chlorophyll—the substance that makes plants green, which is renowned for its cleansing, anti-inflammatory, and rejuvenating properties.

grow your own sprouts

GROWING MY OWN BEAN AND SEED SPROUTS REMINDS ME OF THE EXCITEMENT OF GROWING CRESS AS A SMALL CHILD—ON A BED OF COTTON IN A DARK CUPBOARD. IT'S REMARKABLY EASY AND A REWARDING WAY TO GROW SOME OF YOUR OWN FOOD—ESPECIALLY FOR ANYONE WHO IS A FRUSTRATED, GARDENLESS GARDENER. YOU CAN BUY SPECIALLY DESIGNED TRAYS AND JARS FOR GROWING SPROUTS FROM HEALTHFOOD STORES, BUT HERE'S A SIMPLE ALTERNATIVE.

*about 2 heaped tbsp **seeds**, such as alfalfa, broccoli, radish, or sunflower, or mung or azuki beans*

Punch several holes in the lid of a large, clean jar with a skewer. Put your chosen seeds into the jar. Use just one type per jar, as they grow at different rates. Soak the seeds in plenty of water overnight.

In the morning, drain out the water and rinse the seeds with fresh water, again draining out as much water as possible.

Put the jar in a dark cupboard. Each night and morning, rinse and drain the seeds again until they have sprouted and grown little roots.

After 3–6 days, depending on the type of seed and the warmth, the sprouts will be ready to eat. Once they are ready you can store them in the refrigerator for up to 4 days, but throw them out if they start to turn brown any sooner.

Use in salads or just as a snack. If they have developed little leaves, as broccoli and alfalfa will, leave them on a windowsill for half a day to turn the leaves green before you refrigerate them.

wonderfoods green salad

WITH SO MANY WONDERFUL INGREDIENTS AVAILABLE, THERE'S NO EXCUSE FOR
SERVING A MUNDANE GREEN SALAD BASED ON THE UBIQUITOUS ICEBERG LETTUCE.
THE TASTES AND TEXTURES IN THIS SALAD ARE AMAZING.

*2 handfuls of baby **spinach**
leaves*
*handful of **dandelion** leaves*
*handful of **watercress***
*1 thin slice of **cabbage**,
shredded*
*handful of whatever
sprouts you have*
*1/3 English **cucumber**, sliced*
*3 **scallions**, trimmed and
sliced*
*1 **avocado**, peeled, pitted,
and chopped*
*1 heaped tbsp **pumpkin
seeds***
FOR THE DRESSING
1 heaped tsp Dijon mustard
*1 small **garlic** clove, peeled
and crushed*
*1 tbsp cider vinegar or
balsamic vinegar*
3 tbsp olive oil
fine sea salt
freshly ground black pepper

Trim and wash the spinach, dandelion, and
watercress leaves, pat dry, and place in a large
bowl with the cabbage, sprouts, cucumber,
scallions, and avocado.

To make the dressing, shake the mustard,
garlic, and vinegar together in a lidded jar. Add the
olive oil and a little salt and pepper, and shake again.

Dress the salad just before you eat it and
sprinkle with the pumpkin seeds. It goes
wonderfully with grilled fish or meat.

skin

We spend a lot of time and money nourishing, beautifying, and treating our skin from the outside—with moisturizers and all those creams that promise to reduce the signs of aging. But your skin's best chances may lie in your kitchen. You can slap on all the moisturizer you like, but if you are not feeding your skin the right nutrients, it's going to remain a Sisyphean task!

Dry skin is a common complaint, but just by eating the wonderfoods in this chapter and throughout the book that contain healthy fats, you can go a long way to "oiling" your skin from the inside out. Fats in nuts, seeds, avocados, and fish can be incorporated into the cell membranes to keep them "moisturized." The second advantage to that is that the cells hold onto water better, leaving them nicely plump. One of the most important things to consume for good skin is water—not a wonderfood as such, but, of course, essential to life. Think grapes rather than raisins—and that's what you want on the surface of your body, not to mention your internal "skins" such as those in your gut and lungs.

Healthy skin is also dependent on a good supply of nutrients for the new skin cells to multiply in the deep layers and push through to the surface appropriately. Without enough zinc or vitamin A, for example, this won't take place properly, let alone when you need a wound to heal. Vitamins C and E are also fundamental for the structure of healthy skin.

Many skin problems like rashes, eczema, and psoriasis involve inflammation, so nutrients that help counter this, such as healthy fats and vitamins, can help to relieve some of the symptoms. Another contributory factor to certain skin conditions—acne and psoriasis, for example—are congested bowels, so keeping them moving is important.

External factors, not least sun exposure, can also have a significant impact on the health of your skin. We do need our skin to see some sunlight for good health in order for the body to produce vitamin D, for example. However, excessive tanning under harsh sunlight or by artificial means is known to age the skin and even contribute to skin cancer. Also, the condition of your skin is affected by the substances it comes into contact with—cleaning products around the house, for example—as well as the actual skin care products you use. These can trigger allergic reactions or dry out skin. So watch what you do to your skin externally and eat skin-enhancing wonderfoods that nourish you from the inside, to give you glowing skin.

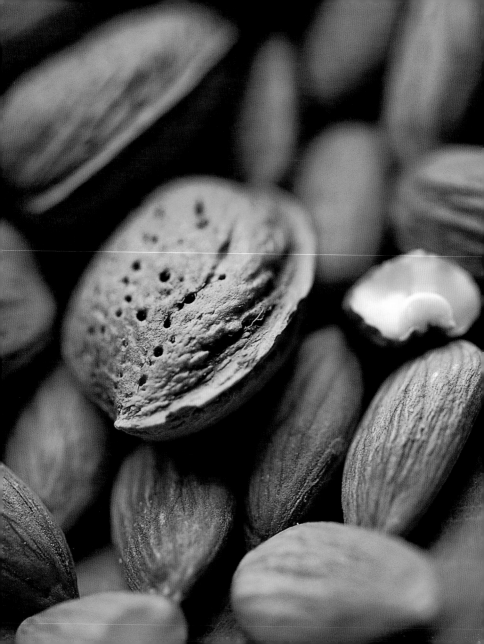

almonds

Nuts are in effect a seed—a concentrated package of goodness waiting to feed a newborn plant as it sprouts—and almonds happen to be one of the best. They are a good source of protein, especially for vegetarians, as well as fiber, B vitamins, vitamin E, calcium, magnesium, iron, and zinc. Almonds have long been used in beauty care, and quite rightly. They are the nut with the highest fiber, which contributes to better elimination of waste products from the body, helping to keep the skin clear. Their vitamin E content plays an important role in skin, inside and out—helping to keep it elastic and to repair it if it is damaged. Almonds also contain monounsaturated fats and plant sterols, both of which help reduce the risk of heart disease. The magnesium in almonds is a useful muscle relaxant and needed to make energy. However, anyone who is susceptible to cold sores or other herpes infections should avoid almonds, as they are rich in the amino acid arginine, which promotes the activation of the virus.

orange almond torte

THIS RICH CAKE IS HEAVENLY—AND YOU CAN FORGIVE YOURSELF ALL THE SUGAR
AND EGGS BECAUSE YOU ONLY NEED A THIN SLICE TO FEEL SATISFIED.

*2 large **oranges***
³/₄ cup + 2 tbsp caster sugar
*2 cups ground **almonds***
*4 **eggs***
*juice of ¹/₂ **lemon***
¹/₂ tsp baking powder

Put the whole, unpeeled oranges in a pan and add cold water to cover. Bring to a boil, then cover and simmer for 2 hours. Drain the oranges and let them cool.

Preheat the oven to 350°F. Grease a 9-inch round cake pan and line with parchment paper. Cut the oranges into chunks and remove the seeds, then tip them into a blender or food processor. Add the remaining ingredients and process until evenly blended. Pour the cake batter into the cake pan. Bake until risen and firm, 45–60 minutes.

Unmold the torte onto a wire rack to cool. It's delicious served warm as a dessert with plain yogurt or sour cream, but equally good eaten cold.

baked stuffed peaches

YOU CAN MAKE AN ALCOHOL-FREE VERSION OF THIS FOR CHILDREN OR
TEETOTALLERS, USING APPLE JUICE INSTEAD OF THE BRANDY.

2 tbsp ground **almonds**
2 amaretti cookies, crushed
2 tbsp brandy
4 ripe peaches, halved and
   pitted
16 **almonds**
$^1/_2$–$^2/_3$ cup **apple** juice

Preheat the oven to 350°F. In a bowl, mix together the ground almonds, crushed cookies, and brandy.

Put the peach halves, skin-side down, in a baking pan. Put a spoonful of the almond mixture into each cavity and top with two almonds. Pour enough apple juice into the dish to cover the bottom, then bake for 30 minutes.

Serve the peaches warm, with plain yogurt, vanilla ice cream, or cream.

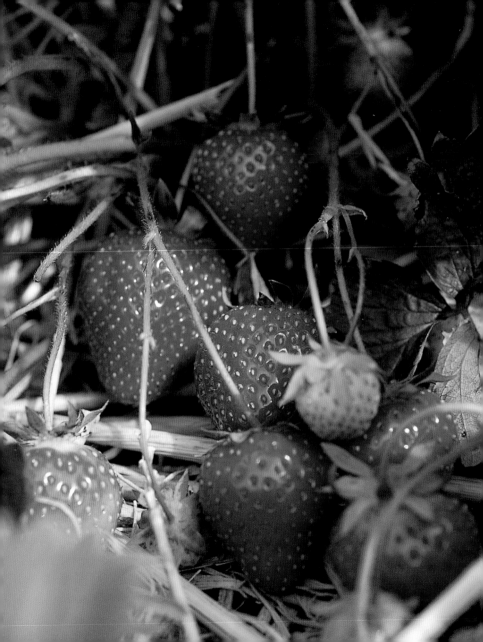

strawberries

It is no coincidence that the Latin name for the world's most popular berry is *fragaria*, referring to its fragrance. And it's not only the taste that is fantastic. Just by eating five strawberries you could obtain half of your recommended daily intake of vitamin C, which is not only needed to protect against colds and cancer, but also for clear skin and skin healing. Strawberries are similarly rich in the lesser-known vitamin K, needed for healthy bones and blood clotting. Their intense color is due to anthocyanin, which protects all the body's cells, including skin, from oxidant damage that contributes to chronic diseases such as heart disease and cancer. Anthocyanins help curb inflammation in conditions like eczema, asthma, and arthritis, too. Another antioxidant in strawberries (and most other berries) that has anti-cancer properties is ellagic acid. The body's own antioxidant enzyme, superoxide dismutase, relies on manganese, which is found in strawberries. The fruit's antioxidants have also been shown to help protect the brain from age-related decline.

artichoke & strawberry salad

I ALWAYS FEEL THERE'S SOMETHING LUXURIOUS ABOUT THIS SALAD THAT BELIES ITS SIMPLICITY. ADJUST THE DRESSING INGREDIENTS TO YOUR TASTE, ADDING A LITTLE MORE ORANGE JUICE, FOR EXAMPLE, IF YOU WANT A MORE TANGY FLAVOR.

large handful of baby
   spinach, *washed*
large handful of arugula
   leaves, washed
4 canned or bottled
   artichoke *hearts in oil,*
   drained and cut into
   pieces
*12 **walnuts***
*8 **strawberries**, sliced*
FOR THE DRESSING
8 medium-large ripe
   strawberries
*1 tbsp **walnut** oil*
*juice of 1/2 **orange***
freshly ground black pepper

To make the dressing, whiz all the ingredients together in a blender until smooth.

Just before serving, combine the spinach and arugula leaves in a salad bowl. Add the artichoke hearts, walnuts, and sliced strawberries, pour the strawberry dressing over, and toss lightly.

appreciating strawberries

I DERIVE A SPECIAL PLEASURE FROM PICKING AND EATING A FRESH STRAWBERRY OFF THE PLANT IN THE GARDEN, ESPECIALLY IF IT'S OF THE SMALL, WILD VARIETY. FOR ME, EVEN CREAM RUINS THE EXPERIENCE OF EATING STRAWBERRIES, SO THERE'S USUALLY NOT MUCH I WANT TO DO TO A FRESH BERRY.

That said, here are a few simple ways of enjoying them:

- Blend with banana, or pretty much any fruit, to make a smoothie for breakfast or a snack.
- Slice and layer with blueberries and plain yogurt.
- Chop and toss with orange juice, cinnamon, and a drop of maple syrup, then roll in a buckwheat crêpe.
- Blend a few strawberries with a little balsamic vinegar and a splash of olive oil to make a salad dressing.

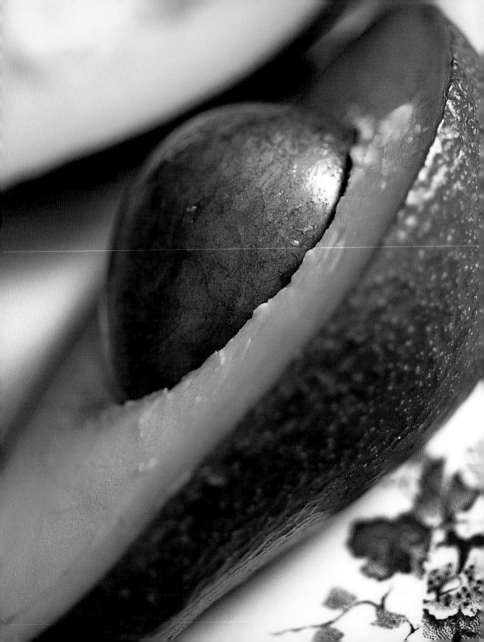

avocado

A member of the laurel family, the avocado tree produces pretty much the most nutritious fruit in the world. The name is derived from the Aztec word for testicle tree, apparently not owing to the shape of the fruit, but because avocados have a reputation for exciting passion! They are loaded with heart healthy monounsaturated fat, fiber, vitamin E, folic acid, iron, niacin, and potassium. Vitamin E is needed to keep the skin soft and supple. As if this was not enough, avocados are also the number one fruit source of beta-sitosterol, a substance that protects against cancer and can reduce total cholesterol. They also surpass other fruits in their content of the antioxidant lutein, which studies have shown helps to protect people from cataracts, cardiovascular disease, and prostate cancer. Avocados are easily digested, and their high fat content means that they are broken down slowly, which is useful for diabetics. They are also one of the richest sources of potassium, which is essential for healthy blood pressure, muscle contraction, and nerve messaging.

avocado red salad

THIS IS A REGULAR IN OUR HOME. YOU COULD ADD SOME CHICKPEAS TO MAKE IT A MORE SUBSTANTIAL SALAD, SUITABLE FOR LUNCH.

handful of shredded red **cabbage**
1 cooked **beet**, peeled and cubed
2 **scallions**, trimmed and finely sliced
handful of shelled young, fresh green peas
1 heaped tbsp chopped **parsley**
2 ripe **avocados**
juice of ½ **lemon**
1 tbsp olive oil
2 tsp tamari or soy sauce
1 heaped tbsp **sunflower seeds**

Put this salad together just before serving. Combine the cabbage, beet, scallions, peas, and chopped parsley in a salad bowl.

Halve, peel, and pit the avocados, then cut into chunks and add to the bowl along with the lemon juice, olive oil, and tamari. Toss gently and scatter the sunflower seeds over.

avocado cream

THIS "SAUCE" TAKES HARDLY ANY TIME TO PREPARE AND GOES WELL WITH PLAIN
GRILLED OR BROILED SEAFOOD, SUCH AS SHRIMP. OR IT CAN BE EATEN AS A DIP
WITH CRUDITÉS AND BREADSTICKS.

2 ripe **avocados**
4 mint leaves
juice of ½ **orange**
juice of ½ **lime**
¼ small red **onion**, peeled
and very finely sliced
pinch of cayenne pepper
pinch of salt
freshly ground black pepper

Halve, peel, and pit the avocados, then tip into a
blender and add the mint, orange juice, lime juice,
and half the onion. Whiz until smooth. Season
with the cayenne, salt, and pepper. Transfer to
a serving bowl and stir in the rest of the onion.
That's it!

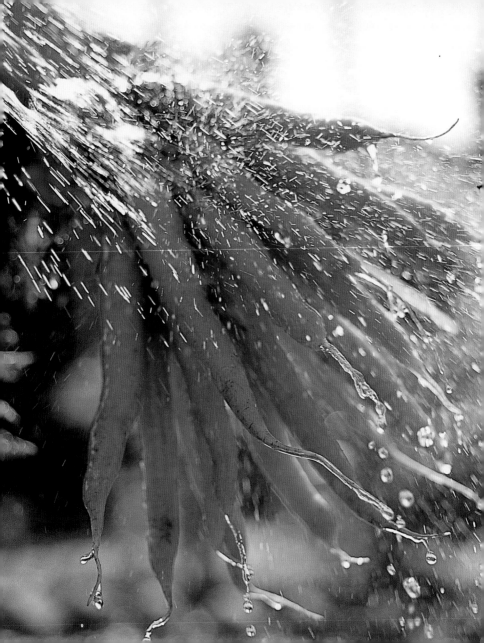

carrot

Ye old faithful carrot—common, inexpensive, versatile, vivid orange, and renowned for helping you see in the dark, although apparently the original carrots from central Asia were purple and not so sweet. Carrots' reputation for helping eyesight is down to their astoundingly high levels of beta-carotene, which the body can convert to vitamin A for use in the skin, gut, and immune system, as well as the eyes. Vitamin A, once in the retina of the eye, is turned into rhodopsin, a purple pigment that's needed for night vision. On top of that, beta-carotene's antioxidant powers help protect against macular degeneration and cataracts. Beta-carotene is just one carotenoid in carrots; another is alpha-carotene, which, with its beta cousin, helps reduce the risk of cancer and heart disease. Carrots are easy to digest, especially when cooked, and loaded with fiber, which is soothing for the digestive tract and boosts detoxification. Another boost for the skin comes from the mineral silica and the vitamin C in carrots.

carrot salad

THIS MAKES AN INTERESTING SIDE SALAD, OR A GREAT LUNCH EATEN SIMPLY WITH A CAN OF TUNA.

*3 medium **carrots**, peeled and grated*
*small handful of shredded **cabbage***
*3 **scallions**, trimmed and finely sliced*
*1 heaped tbsp roughly chopped **parsley***
*small handful of dried **seaweed**, rehydrated*
1–2 tbsp olive oil
*juice of ¹/₂ **lemon***
*1 heaped tbsp toasted **sunflower seeds***

Toss all the ingredients together in a large bowl just before you eat.

carrot & ginger soup

THERE ARE SO MANY VARIATIONS ON THE CARROT SOUP THEME—THIS IS ONE FOR
THOSE WHO LIKE THE HOT TASTE OF GINGER, WHICH CUTS THROUGH THE
SWEETNESS OF THE CARROT PERFECTLY.

1 tsp olive oil
*1 medium **onion**, peeled*
*   and chopped*
*2 **garlic** cloves, peeled*
*   and crushed*
1 tsp mustard powder
*1-inch piece fresh **ginger**,*
*   peeled and grated*
freshly ground black pepper
pinch of salt
4 cups vegetable or chicken
*   stock*
*6 medium-large **carrots**,*
*   peeled and chopped*
*2 **celery** stalks, finely sliced*
2 heaped tbsp roughly
*   chopped **parsley***
*plain **yogurt** for serving*

Heat the olive oil in a large saucepan and soften
the onion and garlic with the mustard powder,
ginger, pepper, and salt, adding 2 or 3 tbsp stock
after a minute or so. After 2–3 minutes longer, add
the carrots and celery, stirring well. Pour in the
rest of the stock and bring to a boil, then cover
and let simmer for about 40 minutes.

When it is ready, whiz the soup until smooth in
a blender, or using an immersion blender in the
pan. Stir in the chopped parsley, saving a little for
garnish, and reheat the soup gently if you need to.

Pour into soup bowls and swirl a spoonful of
yogurt through each portion. Sprinkle with the
reserved chopped parsley and serve.

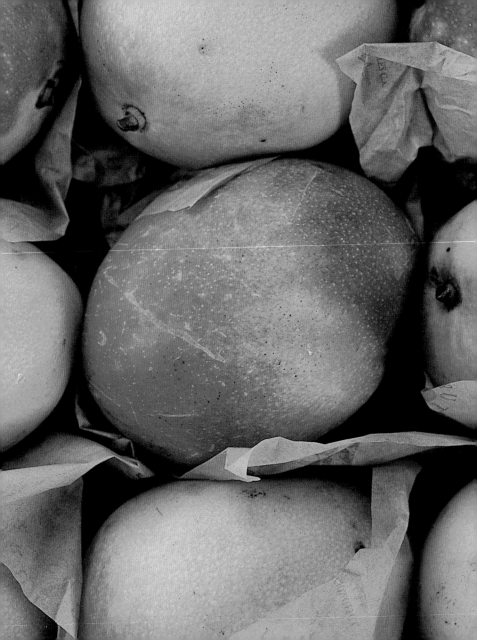

mango

Described by an Indian poet as "sealed jars of honey," mangoes have been cultivated in India for at least 4,000 years. The fragrant, sweet flesh of a juicy mango has to be one of the most sensational taste experiences. And, unlike most sweet delights, mangoes are wonderfully good for you. Their bright orange-yellow color gives away their beta-carotene content. This is the plant form of vitamin A, which is needed for clear, unblemished skin, healthy lungs and intestines, and overall immunity. It complements the vitamin C in the fruit, which is important for the body to produce collagen, a protein in our skin and all connective tissue. Mangoes are a rich source of other antioxidants such as quercetin, which helps protect against allergies and respiratory problems. Like papaya, they contain enzymes that assist the digestion of food and cleansing of the bowel. They are also a good source of iron, potassium, and magnesium, not to mention tryptophan, which the body can convert to the mood hormone, serotonin.

mango & pineapple salsa

I LIKE THIS TANGY, REFRESHING SALSA WITH PLAINLY GRILLED FISH, BUT IT'S ALSO A GREAT WAY TO SPICE UP A TENDER, POACHED CHICKEN BREAST.

2 ripe but firm **mangoes**
1/2 ripe **pineapple**, peeled, cored, and chopped
1/2 red **onion**, peeled and finely sliced
1/2-inch piece fresh **ginger**, peeled and grated
1 **garlic** clove, peeled and crushed
1 small, fresh, hot red chile, finely sliced
handful of cilantro (leaves and stems), roughly chopped
juice of 3 **limes**
2 tsp toasted **sesame** oil

Peel and chop the mangoes over a salad bowl to catch any runaway juice, tipping the fruit into the bowl and discarding the pit. Add the pineapple, onion, ginger, garlic, chile, and cilantro, and toss together. Drizzle with the lime juice and sesame oil, toss to mix, and serve piled on top of grilled fish or chicken.

mango in the buff

AS A CHILD, WHENEVER WE HAD THE LUXURY OF A MANGO, NOT A BIT WAS
WASTED. WE STRIPPED DOWN TO OUR UNDIES, SO AS NOT TO GET IN A MESS, AND
ATE THEM AT A TABLE, FROM WHICH WE COULD EVEN LICK THE JUICE AFTERWARDS!
YOU MAY NOT STRIP TO EAT YOUR MANGOES (NEITHER DO I THESE DAYS), BUT
THEY ARE SO SCENTED AND PRECIOUS, IT'S A SHAME TO ADULTERATE THEM MUCH.
FOR THIS "RECIPE," ALL YOU NEED IS A MANGO AND YOUR TASTEBUDS ON ALERT.

1 *mango*

Firmly squeeze the mango in your hands,
massaging the flesh inside its skin until it feels
soft and separated from the pit. Only then, bite a
small, pea-sized hole in the top and noisily suck
out the molten flesh, squeezing it upward to the
hole. When you really can't get another drop out,
tear back the skin and scrape your teeth along the
inside of each piece. Lastly scrape the pit until
your teeth are filled with shreds of mango hair and
the pit is dry!

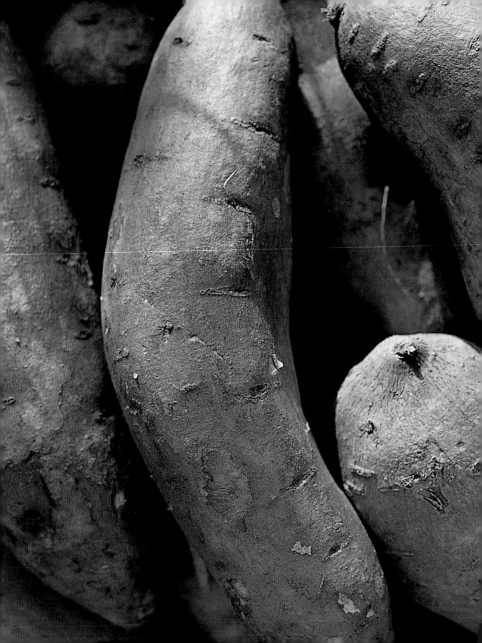

sweet potato

Unrelated to the common potato, the sweet potato is part of the morning glory family and grows on a vine. It is also much more nutritious. There are over 400 varieties, but the orange-fleshed, pink-skinned sweet potatoes—also known by their Maori name *kumara*—are a great source of antioxidants. The more orange, the more abundant is the beta-carotene, the plant form of vitamin A. As such they are beneficial for the skin, eyes, and lungs, and, along with the vitamin C in the vegetable, they provide support for the immune system. The sweetness comes from easily digestible sugars, which makes them a good source of energy, the release of which is somewhat tempered by the fiber content. The easy digestibility means that sweet potatoes are good for any inflammation in the gut, including ulcers. Ideally, cook them in their skins to maximize the conservation of nutrients. Sweet potatoes are wonderfully versatile and can be boiled, baked, roasted, steamed, mashed, and used in both savory and sweet dishes.

sweet potato rösti

THESE RÖSTI ARE GREAT WITH GRILLED SPICED FISH, SUCH AS TUNA OR SARDINES
AND A WONDERFOODS GREEN SALAD (PAGE 111). ALTERNATIVELY, CRUMBLE SOME
GOAT CHEESE INTO AND ON TOP OF THEM AND MAKE SMALLER PATTIES TO SERVE
AS AN APPETIZER, OR MAKE LARGER ONES FOR A VEGGIE MAIN COURSE.

*2 medium **sweet potatoes**,*
  scrubbed
*1 medium **onion**, peeled*
  and grated
*1-inch piece fresh **ginger**,*
  peeled and grated
*1 **egg**, beaten*
fine sea salt
freshly ground black pepper
a little olive oil

Preheat the oven to 400°F. Coarsely grate the
potatoes, then squeeze out as much moisture as
you can, using a kitchen towel. Tip the grated
potatoes into a bowl and mix with the onion,
ginger, egg, salt, and pepper.

Oil a baking sheet with olive oil. Form the
potato mix into four equal patties, about ½ inch
thick, and put them on the oiled sheet. Carefully
turn the patties over (so the tops and bottoms are
both lightly oiled), then bake them until golden
brown and crisp, about 25 minutes.

balsamic baked sweet potatoes

COOKED LIKE THIS, SWEET POTATOES MAKE A GREAT SIDE DISH WITH ANY ROAST
MEAT, CHICKEN, OR FISH, OR THEY CAN BE EATEN AS A MAIN DISH WITH A
TOPPING SUCH AS AVOCADO CREAM (PAGE 127).

*4 small-medium **sweet
potatoes**, scrubbed
2 tbsp balsamic vinegar
4–6 **thyme** sprigs
freshly ground black pepper*

Preheat the oven to 350°F (a slightly higher
temperature is fine if you're using the oven to
roast meat). Toss the sweet potatoes in a baking
dish with 1 tbsp balsamic vinegar and half the
thyme sprigs; season with pepper. Bake until they
feel soft all the way through when tested with a
skewer, about 40 minutes, depending on size.

Slit the potatoes lengthwise, cutting them
halfway through. Drizzle a little balsamic vinegar
into the opening and add a few thyme leaves.

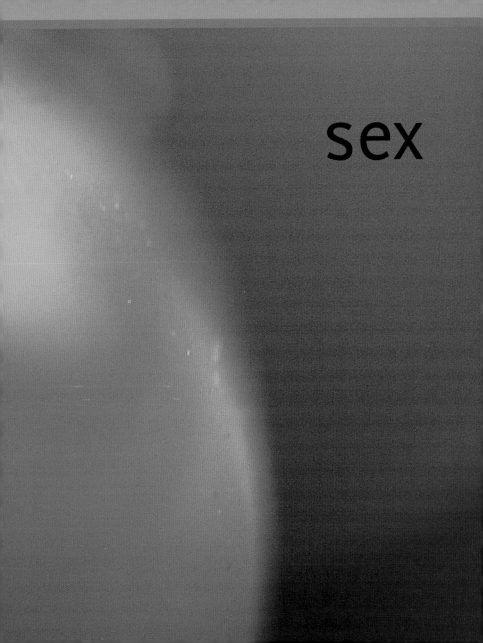

sex

You may want to stop reading now, as I have possibly gotten you to this chapter under a false impression. The wonderfoods herein will not, I'm afraid, acquire you a good sex life or even sex at all (although a nice box of chocolates works for some people, hence its inclusion). There are, however, ingredients here that are known to help fertility and/or hormonal balance in the body.

For many reasons, mainly environmental, dietary, and stress-related, more and more people are finding it difficult to conceive. Obviously, if you are having trouble, working with a professional is a sensible step. Before you get to that stage though, maximizing not only your fertility, but also your chances of conceiving a healthy baby can be done at least in part by optimizing your nutrient intake. Low levels of zinc and vitamin E, for example (both found in seeds), have been linked to infertility. What's more, having good levels of essential nutrients means your body is less likely to hold onto harmful substances like lead, which can interfere with the hormonal system, among others.

Many women who suffer from premenstrual symptoms will give testament to the importance of dietary measures in helping to reduce their monthly pain, cravings, and mood swings. Eating a range of wonderfoods (including small amounts of dark chocolate!) and avoiding caffeine and sugar make a significant difference in relieving such symptoms. Menopausal women also regularly find debilitating symptoms such as hot flushes, night sweats, fatigue, and low moods can be lessened by the careful use of dietary strategies and herbal remedies (best taken under the guidance of a qualified herbalist). Men can benefit from these wonderfoods, too. Increasingly common disorders of the prostate gland have been shown to respond positively to certain nutrients, such as those in pumpkin seeds and tomatoes.

And on a more serious note about sex itself, if you really do find your libido is down, living on a diet of wonderfoods in general, steering clear of foods and drinks that "stress" the body (sugar, caffeine, alcohol, junk food), handling stresses in your life, getting enough sleep, and dealing with any underlying emotional issues—especially with your partner, of course—can go a long way to making you feel horny.

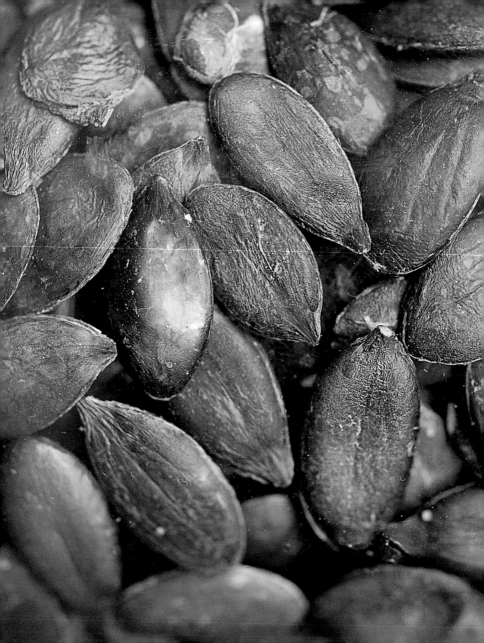

pumpkin seeds

Creamy and nutty, the seeds scooped from your Halloween pumpkin are about the most nutritious and delicious you can buy. They're not only rich in essential fatty acids (EFAs), but also full of important micronutrients, like vitamin E, iron, and magnesium—all needed for good sexual health and fertility. EFAs are important in maintaining smooth, soft, elastic skin that holds water well, so it doesn't become easily dehydrated. The incorporation of EFAs into cell membranes means they are better able to receive hormonal messages. Pumpkin seeds are particularly rich in zinc, a mineral needed for sexual function, defence against infections, proper growth, and the development of new cells. Zinc and EFAs have been linked to helping reduce prostate enlargement. The calcium and magnesium in pumpkin seeds are needed for healthy bones, nerves, and muscles, while the cucurbitacins they contain have anti-inflammatory and anti-cancer properties. Pumpkin seeds are a good source of protein for vegetarians and contain vitamin B_6, which has countless roles, including helping hormone balance in women.

green light salad

THIS IS A STAPLE GREEN SALAD IN OUR HOUSEHOLD, WITH OTHER GREENS FROM THE GARDEN ADDED IN SUMMER, SUCH AS ARUGULA, SORREL, AND LOVAGE. YOU CAN EVEN THROW IN SOME HAZELNUTS OR CHICKPEAS TO MAKE IT A SUBSTANTIAL LUNCH IN ITS OWN RIGHT.

2 handfuls of baby **spinach**, washed
2 handfuls of **watercress**, trimmed and washed
10–12 **basil** leaves
2 **scallions**, trimmed and finely sliced
1 heaped tbsp **pumpkin seeds**
1 **avocado**, peeled, pitted, and chopped
1 tbsp olive oil
juice of ½ **lemon**

Toss all the ingredients together in a large bowl and eat immediately. Or, assemble the leaves, scallions, and pumpkin seeds in advance, adding the avocado, olive oil, and lemon juice at the last minute.

seed-crusted monkfish in prosciutto

BECAUSE OF THE LIGHT MEATINESS OF MONKFISH, IT CAN EASILY CARRY THE
FLAVORS OF OILY PUMPKIN SEEDS AND SALTY HAM.

$^1/_3$ cup **pumpkin seeds**
2 **shallots**, peeled and
    quartered
12 **basil** leaves (or more)
juice of 1 **lemon**
4 pieces of **monkfish** fillet,
    each about 5 oz
4 slices of prosciutto

Preheat the oven to 350°F. Using a mortar and pestle, grind the pumpkin seeds with the shallots, basil, and lemon juice to a rough paste.

Wrap each piece of monkfish in a slice of prosciutto and place in a baking dish. Smear the tops with the seed paste. Pour a little water into the dish, just enough to cover the bottom thinly. Bake until the fish is cooked through, 15–20 minutes. Serve with a salad or steamed green vegetables.

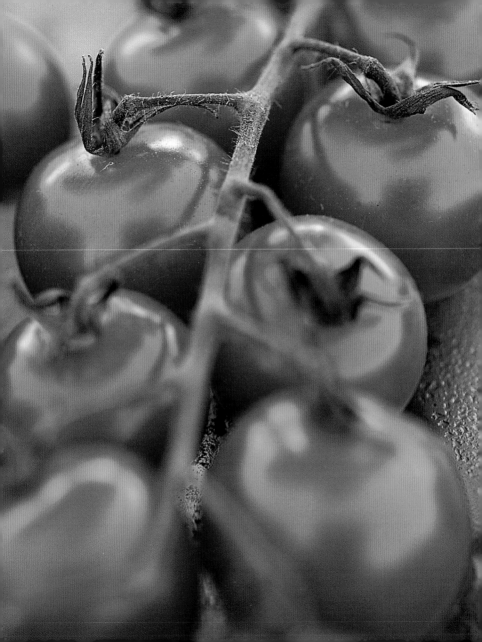

tomato

Originally from the lowlands between the Andes and the Pacific Ocean, the tomato is one of the most commonly eaten wonderfoods. Unlike many fruits and vegetables, some of the benefits of tomatoes are increased when they are cooked. This is because the heating process helps release certain nutrients, notably lycopene, phytoene, and phytofluene—carotenoids that give tomatoes their red color and protective powers. Lycopene has been shown to protect against cancer (especially prostate) and guard the skin and eyes from sun damage. As these carotenoids are fat soluble, they need to be eaten with a little fat to be absorbed (tomatoes with olive oil, for example). The rich vitamin C and potassium content of tomatoes makes them helpful in combating cardiovascular disease. But this fruit has not always been recognized as beneficial to health. Several herbal treatises in the 16th to 19th centuries pronounced the tomato "injurious" and "unwholesome," possibly because, like bell peppers and eggplants, tomatoes contain solanine, which in some people exacerbates the symptoms of arthritis.

frittata tricolore

NAMED AFTER THE ITALIAN FLAG, THIS FRITTATA CAN BE EATEN HOT AS SOON AS IT'S COOKED, OR COLD. YOU'LL NEED A FRYING PAN THAT IS SUITABLE TO USE BRIEFLY UNDER THE BROILER.

6 **eggs**
freshly ground black pepper
splash of olive oil
handful of **spinach**, washed
    and roughly chopped
2 medium **tomatoes**, sliced
4–6 **basil** leaves, torn
5 oz goat cheese, sliced

Preheat the broiler. Beat the eggs in a bowl with some pepper.

Heat the olive oil in a large frying pan over moderate heat, then pour in the beaten eggs. Scatter the spinach, tomatoes, basil, and goat cheese over the egg. Cook for about 3 minutes without stirring, then put the pan under the broiler to cook for a minute or so until the top is golden brown. Serve with a Sunny salad (page 218).

warm chickpea & tomato salad

THIS MAKES A GREAT MAIN COURSE IN ITSELF, OR YOU CAN SERVE IT WITH
A MIDDLE-EASTERN DISH, SUCH AS CARROT FELAFEL (PAGE 183), AS WELL AS
A WONDERFOODS GREEN SALAD (PAGE 111).

1 tbsp olive oil, plus extra
    for drizzling
1 red **onion**, peeled and
    finely sliced
3 **garlic** cloves, peeled
    and sliced
2 tsp grated fresh **ginger**
1 tsp ground cumin
freshly ground black pepper
$1/8$ tsp sea salt
2 cans (14 oz each)
    chickpeas, drained
4–5 tbsp water
1 lb cherry **tomatoes**
4 oz baby **spinach** leaves,
    washed
plain **yogurt** for serving

Heat the olive oil in a large pan and toss in the
onion, garlic, ginger, cumin, pepper, and salt.
Sauté for about 5 minutes, then add the chickpeas
and water. Stir well until most of the liquid has
evaporated, then add the tomatoes and let cook
for 3–4 minutes. Throw in the spinach leaves and
cook briefly until wilted.

Drizzle with a little more olive oil and serve
with plain yogurt to dollop on top. Accompany
with whole-wheat pita bread or brown rice.

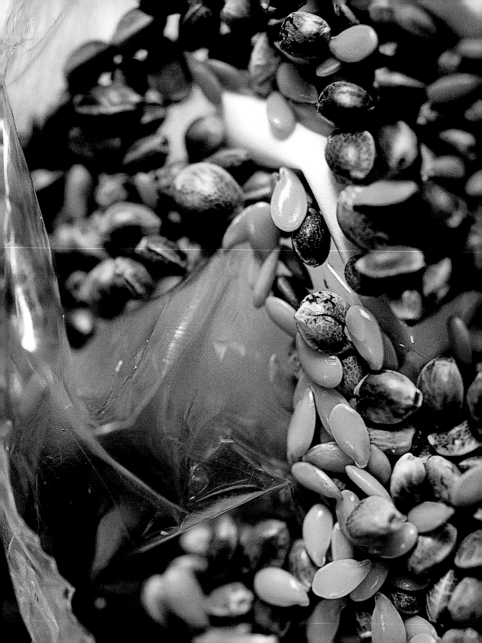

hemp seeds &
flax seeds

If you think these seeds are simply bird food, think again. Both hemp seeds and flax seeds are loaded with omega-6 and omega-3 essential fatty acids (EFAs). These are needed for brain and nerve cells, and therefore important for pretty much all of our body functions, including memory and good moods. Hemp seeds are one of the richest plant sources of omega-3 fatty acids, which help keep blood from clotting excessively, and because of their anti-inflammatory properties, they are natural painkillers—useful for conditions like arthritis. Hemp seeds are also one of the only food sources of GLA, an omega-6 derivative prized for staving off PMS. Flax seeds (also known as linseed) contain lignans, which have been linked to a lower risk of breast and prostate cancers. Like other seeds, hemp and flax seeds contain zinc, calcium, and magnesium. To benefit from their nutrients, it's best to grind them in a coffee grinder, otherwise they won't be digested. Or, to relieve constipation, soak a tablespoonful of flax seeds in a glass of water for a few hours, then drink it down.

high five mix

THIS BLEND OF SEEDS, ONCE GROUND UP, CAN BE USED TO PUT A HEALTHY, NUTTY TOPPING ON YOGURT, CEREAL, SOUPS, AND CASSEROLES. YOU WILL NEED TO KEEP THE SEEDS IN SEALED JARS IN THE REFRIGERATOR, AS THE ESSENTIAL FATTY ACIDS (EFAs) THEY CONTAIN ARE EASILY "DAMAGED" OR OXIDIZED BY HEAT AND LIGHT.

equal quantities of:
flax seeds,
pumpkin seeds,
sunflower seeds,
sesame seeds,
hemp seeds

Grind a batch of mixed seeds in a coffee grinder—kept solely for the purpose, of course! You can do this in advance if you like, provided you keep the ground mix in an airtight jar in the refrigerator. Once crushed, the seeds are even more susceptible to turning rancid, so use within 2–3 weeks.

Scatter the seed mix over yogurt, cereal, soups, or casseroles—to add creaminess and goodness.

toasty seed snack

THIS IS A GREAT SNACK THAT CHILDREN WILL LOVE TOO. YOU CAN ALSO SCATTER IT OVER SALADS TO ADD CRUNCH. MAKE UP A BIG BATCH IN ADVANCE AND STORE IT IN AN AIRTIGHT CONTAINER.

3 heaped tbsp **pumpkin seeds**
3 heaped tbsp **sunflower seeds**
2 heaped tbsp **sesame seeds**
2 heaped tbsp **flax seeds**
1 tbsp tamari or soy sauce

Preheat the oven to 325°F. Line a baking sheet with parchment paper.

In a bowl, toss all the seeds together with the tamari so they are well coated. Scatter the seeds on the lined baking sheet. Toast in the oven for 15 minutes, shaking the sheet or stirring the seeds well a couple of times during cooking.

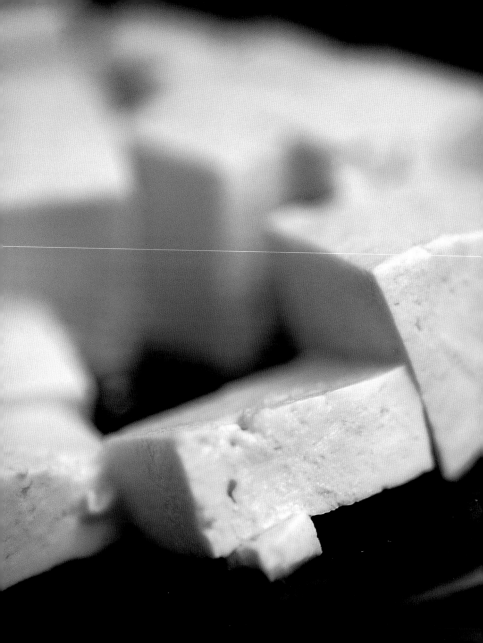

soy

Even if you're not vegetarian, you may well have soy in your diet in some form—perhaps tofu, soymilk, miso, or tempeh. Soymilk is invaluable for those with a sensitivity to cow's milk; some babies are fed on soy-based formulas. For vegans and vegetarians, soy is a good source of first-class protein—containing all the essential amino acids. It is also one of the richest natural sources of isoflavones, a type of phyto (plant) estrogens. These are believed to help block the effect of hormone-disrupting chemicals in our environment, thought to cause problems such as premenstrual syndrome, polycystic ovaries, and breast and prostate cancers. Phytoestrogens may also help if a woman is low in estrogen, for example at the menopause, when they can help to relieve symptoms. Other potential benefits are lowered cholesterol and a reduced risk of osteoporosis. Some studies suggest soy to be harmful, but two or three servings a week is fine, and probably good for you. Buy organic, to avoid genetically modified soy.

roast chicken noodle soup

THIS IS A WONDERFUL DISH TO MAKE WITH LEFTOVER CHICKEN OR DUCK. YOU COULD USE RICE NOODLES INSTEAD OF SOBA, IF YOU PREFER.

2 boneless **chicken** breast halves (with skin)
2 tsp Chinese five spice powder
1 tbsp sweet chile sauce
5 cups water
3 rounded tbsp miso **(soy** paste)
1-inch piece fresh **ginger** or galangal, sliced
2 fresh, hot red chiles, seeded and sliced
2 lemongrass stalks, sliced
5 oz dried soba **(buckwheat)** noodles
2 **scallions**, trimmed and sliced
juice of ½ **lime**
2 handfuls of **mung bean sprouts** (see page 110)
2 heaped tbsp cilantro leaves, torn

Preheat the oven to 350°F. Smear the chicken breasts with the five spice powder and sweet chile sauce, then place in a small roasting pan and roast until they are cooked through, about 25 minutes.

Meanwhile, bring the water to a boil in a large pan. Turn the heat down to a simmer. Scoop out half a mugful and stir the miso paste into this, then pour it back into the pan.

Crush the ginger, chiles, and lemongrass using a mortar and pestle, then add to the soup (or you can just throw them in sliced). Simmer for about 15 minutes, then add the soba noodles, scallions, and lime juice. Cook until the noodles are just tender, 6–8 minutes.

Meanwhile, slice the chicken into bite-sized pieces. Ladle the soup into warm bowls and divide the chicken and mung sprouts among them. Scatter the cilantro over and serve.

sesame tofu stir-fry

I LIKE TO EAT THIS STIR-FRY ON A PILE OF RICE NOODLES THAT HAVE BEEN TOSSED WITH TOASTED SESAME OIL AND CILANTRO LEAVES.

8 oz firm **tofu**, cubed
1 tbsp soy sauce
1/2-inch piece fresh **ginger**, peeled and finely sliced
1 **garlic** clove, peeled and finely sliced
1 tbsp sweet chile sauce
splash of toasted **sesame** oil
4 **scallions**, trimmed and chopped
1 red **bell pepper**, cored, seeded, and cut into strips
1 **carrot**, peeled and cut into thin strips
handful of snow peas
2–3 tbsp water
1 heaped tbsp finely chopped cilantro leaves
2 heaped tbsp **sesame seeds**

Put the tofu in a bowl with the soy sauce, ginger, garlic, and chile sauce. Toss to mix, then set aside to marinate while you prepare the vegetables.

Heat a wok or large frying pan and add a splash of sesame oil. Add the tofu along with its marinade and toss continuously over high heat for a couple of minutes. Remove the tofu with a slotted spoon and set aside on a plate.

Add the scallions, red pepper, carrot, and snow peas to the wok. Toss quickly, and then add 2–3 tbsp water to "steam-fry" the vegetables. Stir well over high heat for about 2 minutes.

Add the chopped cilantro. Put the tofu back into the pan to reheat briefly, but don't let the vegetables become too soft. Sprinkle the stir-fry with sesame seeds and serve.

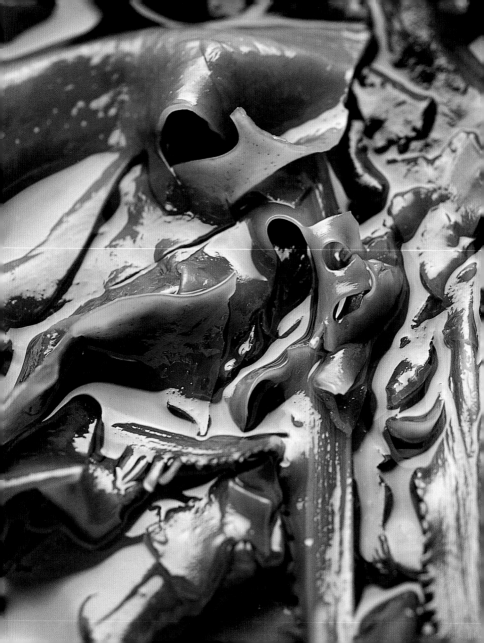

seaweed

It's the wafting weed that gives you the creeps as it brushes your leg in the sea, but seaweed is one of nature's true wonderfoods and it has been eaten for millennia—you will find it depicted in Egyptian hieroglyphs. Wild seaweed, or algae, is a great source of minerals and a powerful cleanser, as long as it hasn't been harvested from polluted waters. It's a very good source of iodine, which is an important player in the body's hormonal system. This mineral is needed to make the thyroid hormone that is responsible for dictating our body's metabolism, i.e. all its activities. An underactive thyroid is linked to fatigue and a low sex drive. The chlorophyll that makes seaweed green is a natural detoxifier and its alginic acid helps draw out waste. Seaweed also contains lignans, which have cancer-protective properties, and it provides the full alphabet of essential minerals and vitamins—in a natural balance that enhances the synergy of the nutrients. We would all do well to include seaweed in our diet regularly.

crunchy summer salad

YOU CAN ADD SOME SHREDDED CABBAGE TO MAKE THIS SALAD EVEN CRUNCHIER.
SERVE IT AS A LIGHT FIRST COURSE, OR AS A SIDE DISH WITH NOODLES OR A STIR-FRY.

small handful of dried
seaweed, *such as arame*
3 medium-large **carrots**,
peeled and grated
3 **scallions**, *trimmed and*
finely sliced
about 10 cilantro sprigs,
roughly chopped
2 tsp toasted **sesame** *oil*
1 tbsp tamari or soy sauce
juice of 1–2 **limes**, *to taste*
1 heaped tbsp **sesame seeds**

Put the seaweed in a mug, pour in just enough boiling water to cover, and let steep for 4–5 minutes. Meanwhile, in a large bowl, combine the carrots, scallions, and cilantro.

When the seaweed is soft, drain it in a strainer, tossing to cool it off before adding to the salad. Add the sesame oil, tamari, and lime juice (using more rather than less if you want a tangy flavor). Toss all the ingredients together well.

Just before serving, sprinkle the sesame seeds over the salad.

enjoying seaweed

IF YOU'RE NOT USED TO COOKING WITH SEAWEED, THE IDEA MAY INITIALLY SEEM
A BIT DAUNTING, BUT IT IS REMARKABLY VERSATILE AND TASTY... NOT TO MENTION
BEING A WONDERFOOD.

- Healthfood stores and wholefood markets now sell a range of dried
  Japanese varieties, such as wakame, hijiki, and arame. These need
  rehydrating before use and can be added to soups, stir-fries, stews, or salads.
- You can also get dried seaweeds from the Pacific and Atlantic coasts, such
  as dulse, laver, and sea lettuce. Specialist fish merchants sometimes sell
  them fresh or non-dried, usually preserved in salt or pickled. Rinse these
  well and eat them raw in salads, stir-fries, omelets, or soups.
- Seaweed the windbreaker: When you're cooking dried beans or chickpeas,
  add a strip of kombu, a Japanese seaweed. It helps reduce the wind factor in
  the beans by making them more easily digestible.

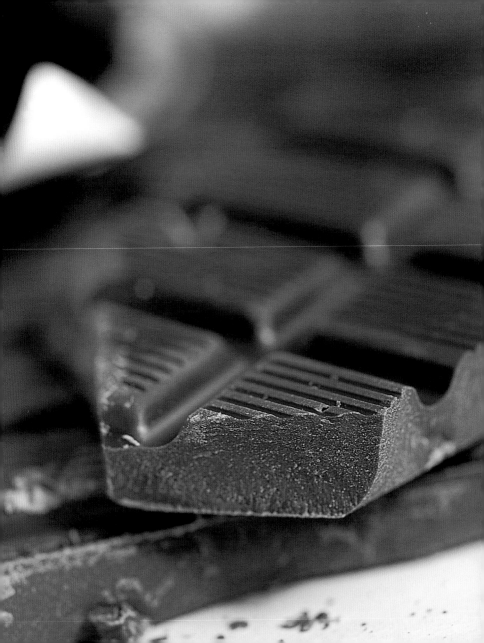

chocolate

It is said the Aztec emperor Montezuma drank chocolate daily to enhance his sexual prowess, though it would have been a very different drink from today. There's no clear reason why chocolate is considered sexy or romantic, but the rich, sweetness blended with a light stimulant may be what makes it a lovers' favorite. Its divine properties are acknowledged in its classification: *Theobroma cacao*—theobroma meaning food of the gods. Chocolate's major ingredient, cocoa, is a source of theobromine, which mildly stimulates the nervous system. Chocolate contains small amounts of mood-enhancing phenethylamine, too. It also has a high content of antioxidants, including polyphenolic flavonoids, which reduce inflammation, keep blood vessels healthy, and lower the risk of cancer. That said, regular consumption of fats and sugars in chocolate is linked to health problems. So eat organic, dark chocolate, which contains more cocoa and therefore less sugar and fat. Chocolate is good for the soul and that makes it a wonderfood in my book!

baked banana-choc split

THIS RECIPE CAN EVEN BE COOKED ON THE GRILL—THE FIRST TIME I MADE IT WAS UNDER A GLORIOUSLY STARRY NIGHT ON A BEACH IN SOUTH DEVON IN ENGLAND. IT COULDN'T BE EASIER.

4 **bananas** (unpeeled)
12 small squares of dark,
     organic **chocolate**
4 heaped tbsp sour cream
16 **almonds**, roughly
     broken up

Preheat the oven to 350°F. Lay the bananas, still in their skins, on a baking sheet and bake until they are soft, 20–25 minutes.

Lay each banana on its side on a plate and make a slit along most of the length, through the skin and halfway through the banana. Squeeze the slit open by pushing up from the outside of the skin. Slip 3 pieces of chocolate into each slit and spoon on the sour cream.

Top with the almonds and serve immediately, as the chocolate melts.

chocolate refrigerator slice

CHILDREN WILL LOVE MAKING—AND EATING—THIS ONE. BIG CHILDREN TOO! YOU CAN USE ANY DRIED FRUIT YOU FANCY.

1/4 cup **almonds**, roughly broken up
3 heaped tbsp **pumpkin seeds**
5 oz dried fruit, such as raisins, **apricots, papaya, berries**
1/4 cup brandy (or orange juice)
6 oz dark, organic **chocolate**
3 1/2 tbsp unsalted butter
3 oz graham crackers (5 large rectangles), broken into small pieces

If you want to roast the almonds and pumpkin seeds to enhance their flavor, toss them in a dry frying pan for a few minutes until they brown a little and the pumpkin seeds pop. Let cool.

Cut larger dried fruits into small, raisin-sized pieces. Put all the fruit in a bowl, add the brandy, stir well, and set aside to macerate.

Line an 8-inch tart or cake pan with plastic wrap, letting it hang over the rim. Melt the chocolate and butter together in a small pan over very low heat—take care to avoid overheating.

Drain the dried fruit and return to the bowl. Mix in the almonds, pumpkin seeds, and graham crackers. Add the melted chocolate mixture and stir it all together well. Pour into the prepared pan and refrigerate overnight until firm. Serve in slices, as it is or with a little sour cream.

age

It won't come as any surprise that I'm not suggesting eating the foods in this section will turn back the clock for you, or enable your liver to cope with partying as you did when you were twenty! But there are legitimate, scientific reasons why these foods all fall under the age category of wonderfoods. They are all particularly high in naturally occurring chemicals with antioxidant properties.

Antioxidants counter the effect of oxidants, which are sometimes known as free radicals. Oxidants are highly reactive compounds that are produced when the body uses oxygen. The body has very sophisticated mechanisms in the form of antioxidant enzyme systems to go around mopping up after the oxidants. We are also exposed to oxidants in our environments, from car exhaust fumes, pesticides, sun radiation, smoking, alcohol, some medications, and even charred food.

Although oxidants are normal by-products of the body's workings and our surroundings, there is no doubt that excessive exposure is detrimental to health, particularly when coupled with insufficient exposure to antioxidants. In effect, oxidants multiply through a chain reaction, creating a cascade of damage, particularly to cell membranes and our cell reproductive blueprint, our DNA. Scientists have made clear links between oxidants and several degenerative diseases (such as heart disease, cancer, Alzheimer's) and the aging process. Also linked to aging is a decline in the body's immune system and a higher risk of infection; antioxidants can also help support immunity.

Common antioxidants are vitamins A, C, and E, beta-carotene, selenium, zinc, and flavonoids. A good daily dose of these protective substances is crucial for good health and to minimize the aging process. I'm not necessarily referring to ironing out those crow's feet or frown lines, but more the internal aging of our bodies that leaves them not working quite as efficiently as they used to. And no amount of these foods is going to compensate for the set of genes you were born with, as well as habits like smoking or other factors that contribute to aging. The foods in this category need to be eaten alongside others throughout the book and even then, your diet is just one thing to consider in helping you age gracefully and in good health. Others are: getting sufficient sleep, exercizing appropriately, and not overeating. Whatever else you do, as long as you're eating good amounts of the foods in this section and other wonderfoods, at least you're maximizing your chances of minimizing aging.

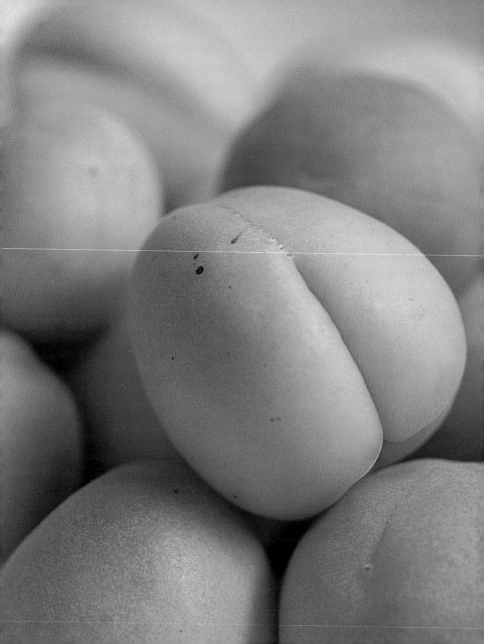

apricot

The softness of a ripe apricot may not yield the juiciest of flesh, but it certainly packs a punch with flavor and health. It is even said to have been the original nectar of the gods. Like other orange-colored fruit and vegetables, apricots are a mine of beta-carotene, which protects the skin and lungs from oxidation damage and supports a healthy immune system. Apricots are rich in fiber, so they can help relieve constipation and ward off digestive problems such as diverticulitis, particularly when eaten dried. Too much dried fruit, though, can cause bloating, so stop yourself from eating too many—you probably wouldn't eat ten fresh apricots, so best not to eat ten dried ones all at once! Although fresh apricots are best eaten either alone, in smoothies or desserts, the dried ones make an interesting addition to savory meat or chicken dishes, as they are used in the Middle East. Most dried apricots are preserved with sulfur dioxide, so go for the darker, non-sulfured ones.

spiced apricots

THIS IS ONE OF THE MOST POPULAR, EASY, AND HEALTHY DESSERTS I MAKE. IF YOU HAVE A PACKAGE OF DRIED APRICOTS IN THE CUPBOARD, YOU CAN RUSTLE IT UP AT SHORT NOTICE FOR GUESTS.

7 oz dried **apricots**
1 cup water
¹/₂ cup **apple** *juice*
3 star anise
10 **cardamom** *pods*

Put all the ingredients in a saucepan and bring to a boil. Cover and let simmer for at least an hour to get the most out of the spices, though less will do if you don't have the time. Take the lid off if you want to reduce the syrup further.

Serve with plain yogurt or, if you're feeling more indulgent, vanilla ice cream.

apricot salsa

THIS FRESH, RAW "CHUTNEY" GOES PERFECTLY WITH CHEESE AND ALL SORTS OF
SAVORY DISHES, SUCH AS CARROT FELAFEL (PAGE 183) AND PLAIN ROAST OR
GRILLED CHICKEN AND MEAT. MAKE SURE THE APRICOTS ARE NICELY RIPE TO
SWEETEN THE WHOLE MIX.

6 ripe **apricots**, pitted and
    finely chopped
1 heaped tbsp capers,
    roughly chopped
2 **shallots** (or 1 small red
    onion), peeled and very
    finely diced
few **basil** leaves, roughly
    torn
juice of 1 **lemon** (or ½ if
    it's large)
pinch of ground **cinnamon**
2 tbsp olive oil
freshly ground black pepper

Mix all the ingredients together in a bowl. Ideally,
leave for about an hour to let the flavors infuse,
although the salsa still tastes fine if you serve it
right away.

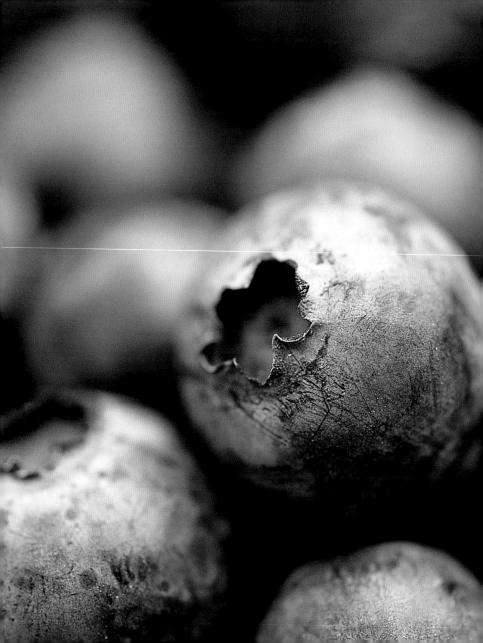

blueberries

Native Americans have known for centuries that juicy blueberries are remarkable. Sometimes called bilberries, they are an amazing source of antioxidants, particularly anthocyanidins, as are another dark relative, blackberries. These potent chemicals are protective in their own right against aging caused by oxidant damage, but also help increase the potency of vitamin C. Studies have shown that blueberries can help to improve brain function and they have an affinity with the eyes, helping night vision and protecting against age-related macular degeneration, cataracts, and glaucoma. Blueberries strengthen the entire vascular system (veins and arteries), making sure that all parts of the body get sufficient oxygen and vital nutrients. They also contain a substance called pterostilbene, which helps lower cholesterol and protect against cancer. The antioxidants in blueberries help protect our cellular support structure, collagen, from oxidant damage—so improving skin tone. Blueberries are also a good source of fiber.

blueberry cheesecake

YOU CAN VARY THIS CHEESECAKE BY USING ALL SORTS OF OTHER FRUIT, SUCH AS
RASPBERRIES, STRAWBERRIES, OR PITTED CHERRIES. IF YOU WANT A GLUTEN-FREE
DESSERT, OMIT THE BASE, MAKE 1½ TIMES THE AMOUNT OF FILLING, SPOON INTO
A BOWL, TOP WITH THE BLUEBERRIES, AND CHILL BEFORE SERVING.

FOR THE BASE
1¼ cups rolled **oats**
6 tbsp chopped **almonds**
1 heaped tbsp brown sugar
    or alternative equivalent
    (see page 10)
1 tsp ground **cinnamon**
⅓ cup butter, melted
FOR THE FILLING
1¼ cups cream cheese
2 tbsp amaretto liqueur
    (or water)
2 tbsp **lemon** juice
2 heaped tbsp confectioners'
    sugar
FOR THE TOPPING
2 cups **blueberries**

Preheat the oven to 350°F. For the base, mix the
oats, almonds, sugar, and cinnamon together
in a large baking pan and toast in the oven for
20–25 minutes. (I sometimes first grind the oats
in a blender for a minute—to make a finer base.)

Meanwhile, prepare the topping. In a bowl, beat
the cream cheese with the amaretto, lemon juice,
and confectioners' sugar until evenly blended.

When the base ingredients are toasted, stir in
the melted butter and press the mixture over the
bottom of a 9-inch tart pan. Ideally, let it set in the
refrigerator for a couple of hours.

Spread the cream cheese mixture over the base
and top with the blueberries. Refrigerate until
ready to serve.

mango incognito

YOU CAN BARELY MAKE OUT THE MANGO FROM THE COLOR OF THIS DELICIOUS
SMOOTHIE, BUT THE TASTE CERTAINLY TELLS YOU IT'S THERE. THE GUAVA ADDS A
DIFFERENT DIMENSION ALTOGETHER, ALTHOUGH YOU CAN USE APPLE IF YOU
CAN'T FIND GUAVA JUICE.

*3 handfuls of **blueberries***
*1 large **mango** (or 2 small ones)*
*1/2 cup plain **yogurt***
*1/2 cup guava juice (or **apple** juice)*

Whiz all the ingredients together in a blender and drink immediately, but not quickly!

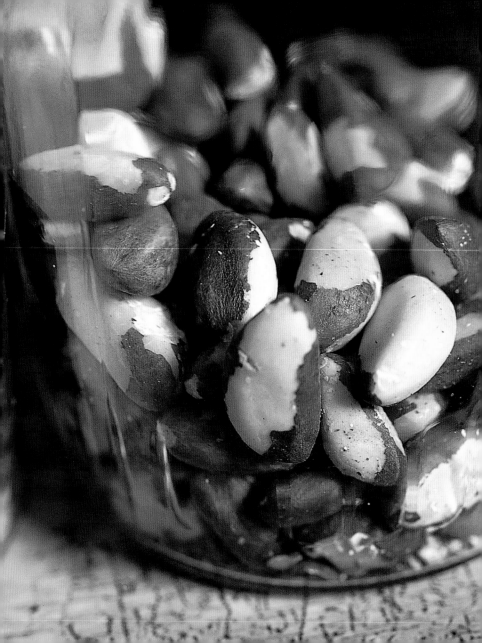

brazil nuts

Unlike much of the food we eat, Brazil nuts have yet to be grown successfully on plantations—they are harvested from huge, wild trees in the Latin American rainforest. The wedge-shaped nuts form segments in fruits that are about the size of a large grapefruit. Nutritionally, Brazil nuts are best known for their rich selenium content. This mineral is needed to activate an enzyme in the body called glutathione peroxidase, which helps protect us against oxidants and the development of cancer cells. Studies have shown that a higher selenium intake is linked to a lower incidence of various types of cancer. Selenium is also needed by the immune system, for thyroid hormones to work properly, and for healthy sperm. Brazil nuts are about 70% fat: half is oleic (as in olive oil) and much of the rest is omega-6 with some omega-3. Because of this, it is best to buy Brazils in their shells, as the fat is prone to turn rancid and the nut keeps better in its natural case.

brazil nut & watercress pesto

THIS DELICIOUS SAUCE NOT ONLY GOES WITH PASTA, LIKE A REGULAR PESTO, BUT ALSO WITH ANY GRILLED FISH OR MEAT.

*16–20 **Brazil nuts**, shelled*
*2 **garlic** cloves, peeled*
2 large handfuls of
   ***watercress**, washed*
5 oz Parmesan cheese,
   finely (and freshly)
   grated (about 1¼ cups)
*juice of ½ **lemon***
freshly ground black pepper
3–4 tbsp olive oil (or more,
   if needed)

Whiz the nuts, garlic, watercress, Parmesan, lemon juice, and a generous grinding of pepper together in a blender, adding the olive oil a little at a time until you have a smooth, fresh sauce.

Toss the pesto with freshly cooked pasta or serve spooned over hot, grilled fish or meat.

carrot felafel

THESE ARE A LESS DENSE VERSION OF MIDDLE-EASTERN CHICKPEA FALAFEL. THEY
ARE GREAT SERVED WITH APRICOT SALSA (PAGE 175), PLAIN YOGURT, AND A
WONDERFOODS GREEN SALAD (PAGE 111), OR ROLLED IN A WARM PITA BREAD
WITH A LITTLE TAHINI (SESAME PASTE), CHILE SAUCE, TOMATOES, AND CUCUMBER.
FOR A VEGETARIAN MAIN COURSE, DOUBLE THE QUANTITIES LISTED.

³/₄ cup **chickpeas** (cooked
  or canned and well
  drained)
1 small **onion**, peeled and
  quartered
1 **garlic** clove, peeled
handful of **parsley**
¹/₂ tsp ground cumin
¹/₂ tsp ground coriander
¹/₂ tsp cayenne pepper (or
  a dash of hot pepper
  sauce)
¹/₂ tsp baking powder
6 **Brazil nuts**, shelled
3 medium **carrots**, peeled
  and grated
4 dried **apricots**, finely
  chopped
1 **egg**, beaten
a little olive oil
FOR SERVING (OPTIONAL)
²/₃ cup plain **yogurt**
squeeze of **lemon** juice
small handful of chopped
  cilantro

Put the chickpeas, onion, garlic, parsley, spices, baking powder, and nuts in a blender and process briefly to a rough paste. Ideally there will still be a few chunks of Brazils. Tip the mixture into a bowl. If you prefer, you can break up the nuts with a mortar and pestle and add them at this stage (rather than earlier).

Add the grated carrots, chopped apricots, and beaten egg and mix thoroughly. Form the mixture into 12 small balls and flatten them slightly.

Spray a nonstick pan with a little olive oil and place over moderate heat. Add the falafel and fry lightly until they're brown on both sides.

Meanwhile, if you are serving it, flavor the yogurt with lemon juice and cilantro to taste. Serve the falafel warm, with the yogurt.

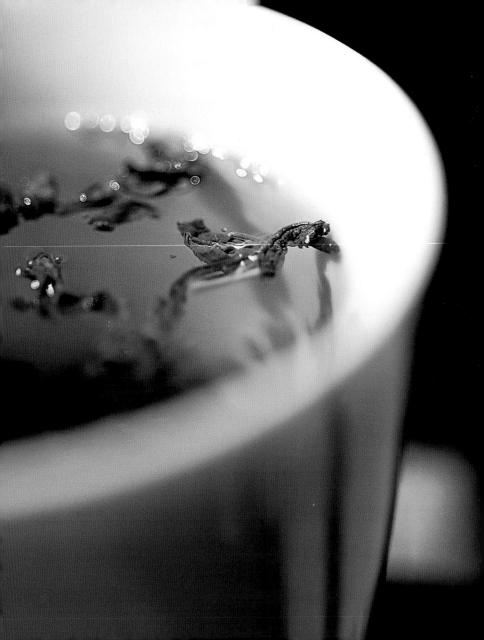

green tea

The leaves for this delicate drink come from the same plant as black tea, but they are lightly steamed when freshly cut, rather than left to dry out and turn black, so more of the goodness is preserved. There are several antioxidant chemicals called flavonoids in green tea that make it so beneficial, but the most effective is thought to be one called epigallocatechin gallate. Oxidants are an inevitable part of life—our bodies even produce them—but pollution, the sun, smoking, smoky atmospheres, and fried foods expose us to even more. An excess of oxidants has been linked to chronic conditions such as heart disease and cancer, as well as accelerated aging. Given that green tea can contain about eight times as much antioxidant power as black tea, a couple of cups a day is certain to offer some protection. Gut-wise, the tannins in tea can help stop diarrhea. Remember though, that green tea does contain some caffeine, which can irritate the gut, stimulate the nervous system, and make you restless.

poached figs

USE EITHER LOOSE LEAVES OR A TEABAG TO MAKE THE GREEN TEA FOR THIS
LOVELY, LIGHT DESSERT, WHICH CAN ALSO BE SERVED AS A SIDE DISH WITH
GRILLED OR ROASTED MEAT.

1¼ cups **green tea**
2 tbsp **honey**
6 **thyme** sprigs, plus extra
   sprigs for serving
½ cup Marsala wine
½ **lemon**, sliced (seeds
   removed)
8 fresh, ripe figs, washed
   and cut in half
plain **yogurt** for serving

In a large saucepan, combine the green tea, honey, thyme, and wine. Bring to a boil, lower the heat, and add the lemon slices. Stir constantly until the honey is completely dissolved.

Halve the figs vertically, add them to the green tea solution, and poach for about 2 minutes on each side. Remove the figs with a slotted spoon and place in serving bowls.

Boil the liquid in the pan until it is syrupy. Drizzle the syrup all over the figs and top each portion with a slice of lemon and some thyme. Serve with yogurt or cream.

green tea refresher

THIS IS A WONDERFUL DRINK ON A HOT SUMMER DAY. YOU CAN USE OTHER TYPES OF FRUIT JUICE—FRESHLY SQUEEZED GRAPEFRUIT IS PARTICULARLY TANGY.

4 cups freshly made
   green tea
2-inch piece fresh **ginger**,
   peeled and grated
small bunch of mint leaves
1 cup **pineapple** juice
lots of ice cubes

Combine the freshly made green tea with the ginger and half the mint in a large pitcher and set aside to cool.

Add the rest of the mint, the pineapple juice, and the ice cubes just before serving and stir well.

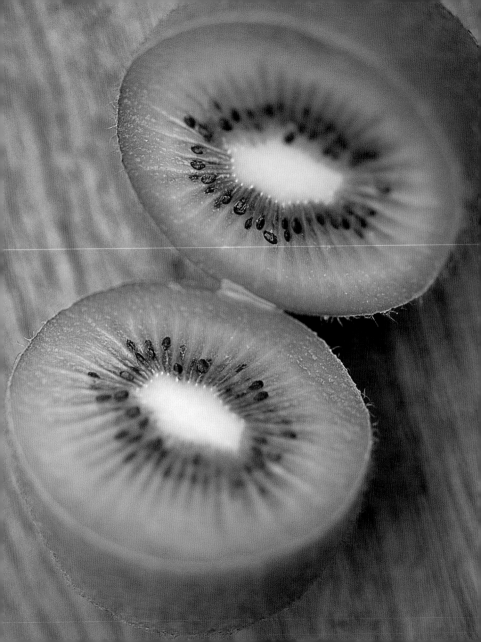

kiwi fruit

New Zealanders renamed the Chinese gooseberry in the 1950s as a marketing strategy, hence the name "kiwi fruit." Still, it beats the original French name of *souris vegetale*, or "vegetable mouse." Whatever you call them, kiwi fruit are, like most foods in this section, loaded with antioxidants, including a member of the carotene family, lutein, as well as vitamins C and E. Scientists have found that eating two or three kiwi fruit a day helps reduce blood clotting (and therefore stroke) potential as well as blood fats. Kiwis are right up there with bananas on the potassium front, so they are good for balancing out your salt intake to keep your blood pressure right. Kiwis are also digestive aids, firstly because they are high in fiber that's useful for blood-sugar control and for helping lower cholesterol, and secondly, because they contain an enzyme called actinidin, which actually helps digest proteins in food—like the enzyme papain in papaya. Beware though, that some people—particularly young children—can have an allergic reaction to kiwi fruit, especially from its skin.

kiwi & figs with prosciutto

I FIRST ATE THIS AT A FRIEND'S HOUSE IN THE SOUTH OF FRANCE. IT'S A SURPRISINGLY WONDERFUL COMBINATION.

*4 ripe **kiwi fruit,** peeled*
4 ripe figs
8 thin slices of prosciutto
splash of balsamic vinegar
    (optional)
splash of olive oil (optional)

Slice the kiwi fruit in half lengthwise and the figs into three from top to bottom. Arrange a fig and a kiwi on each plate, along with two slices of prosciutto.

I don't think there is any need for a dressing here, but if desired, drizzle with a little balsamic vinegar and a splash of olive oil.

pastel perfect kiwi

THIS DELICIOUS SMOOTHIE CAN BE SHARP ON THE TONGUE IF THE FRUITS AREN'T NICE AND RIPE, SO PICK YOUR MOMENT WELL.

$^1/_2$ **pineapple**, *peeled, cored, and roughly chopped*
3 **kiwi fruit**, *peeled*
$^1/_2$ *cup* **pineapple** *juice*

Put all the ingredients in a blender and whiz until smooth. Drink immediately.

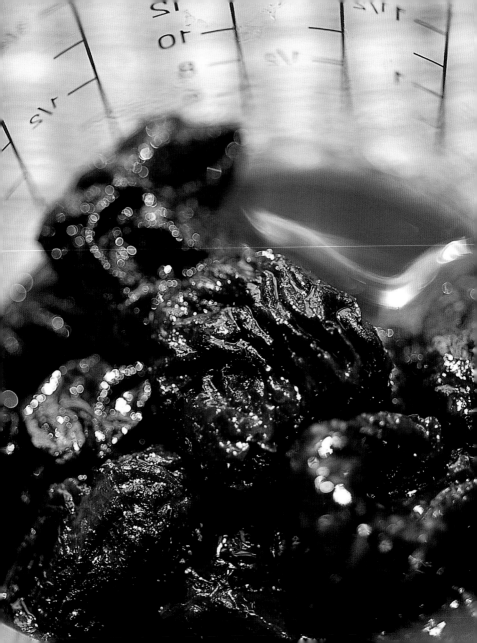

prunes

Prunes have long been recognized as a very rich source of fiber that's good for keeping your bowel movements regular, but there is much more to them than that. Prunes are one of the top foods for total antioxidant power. These vital chemicals in foods are essential for keeping your skin clear, improving your detoxification, protecting you from disease, and generally keeping the inevitable aging process in check. So don't wait until your face looks like a prune to start eating them—even they won't reverse wrinkles. However, scientists have shown that your diet can affect how wrinkly your skin becomes with age. There's more—prunes are fat-free and high in the important minerals potassium and iron. Remember that prunes are dried plums; the two words (the former French, the latter, Anglo-Saxon) were used interchangeably until recent times). So plump, fresh plums are also wonderfoods, just less so than prunes, weight for weight.

moroccan lamb

THIS IS AN ABSOLUTE FAVORITE IN OUR HOME ON A WINTER'S NIGHT—WITH ALL THOSE AROMAS, YOU COULD BE IN MARRAKECH BUT FOR THE COLD OUTSIDE.

10 oz lean, boneless **lamb**
3 **garlic** cloves, crushed
1 heaped tbsp harissa or
    chile paste
juice of 1 **lemon**
freshly ground black pepper
small handful of mint,
    chopped
splash of olive oil
8 **shallots**, peeled
1 **cinnamon** stick
7 **cardamom** pods
2 tsp ground cumin
5 medium-large **tomatoes**,
    peeled and chopped
1½ cups **chickpeas** (cooked
    or canned and drained)
10–12 **prunes**
about 2½ cups water
small handful of cilantro
    leaves, chopped

Cut the lamb into bite-sized cubes. In a bowl, mix the garlic with the harissa, lemon juice, some pepper, and half the mint. Add the lamb, toss to coat, and let marinate while you prepare the other ingredients.

Heat a splash of olive oil in a large saucepan, then add the shallots with the spices and cook, stirring, for a minute or two. Add the lamb, along with its marinade, and stir well for a few minutes until it is lightly browned all over. Add the tomatoes, chickpeas, and prunes, plus the water. Stir well, then cover and let simmer until the lamb is tender, about 1 hour.

Add the remaining mint and the cilantro just before serving. Eat with brown rice or couscous.

drunken prunes

EVEN PEOPLE WHO SAY THEY DON'T LIKE PRUNES LOVE THIS RICH DESSERT.

20–24 **prunes**
$1/2$ cup **apple** juice
$1/2$ cup water
$1/4$ cup brandy
1-inch piece fresh **ginger**,
    peeled and sliced
finely pared zest of
    1 **orange**
10–12 **almonds**, shelled
FOR SERVING
$2/3$ cup plain **yogurt**
$1/2$ tsp vanilla extract, or
    to taste

Put the prunes in a saucepan and add the apple juice, water, brandy, ginger, and orange zest. Bring to a boil, then immediately turn the heat down to a simmer. Cook, uncovered, for 15–20 minutes.

Meanwhile, toast the almonds for a few minutes under a hot broiler, then roughly crush them, using a mortar and pestle or small food processor. Mix the yogurt with the vanilla extract.

Using a slotted spoon, divide the prunes among four bowls. Top each with a dollop of yogurt and drizzle some of the cooking liquid over. Sprinkle with the crushed almonds and serve.

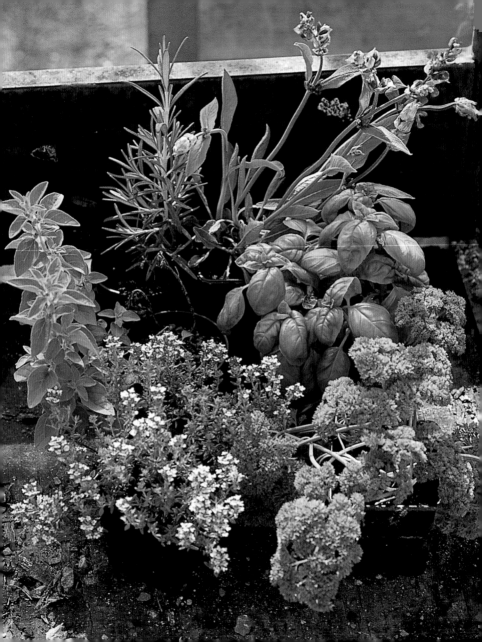

mediterranean
herbs

The scent of fresh, wild thyme being crushed under my feet on Maltese clifftops is a strong childhood memory, but the aroma is just part of the story. Mediterranean herbs—thyme, sage, parsley, oregano, basil, and rosemary—are brimming with health benefits that have been recognized for ages. Herbs were used to help preserve foods, to protect them from microbial contamination, and now research has shown that they protect us, too. All, but especially oregano, contain chemicals that kill infectious microbes. Thymol, an oil in thyme leaves, is powerfully antiseptic and good for coughs and chest infections. It also helps protect the fats found in cell membranes, particularly the brain and heart, from oxidant damage and therefore rapid aging. Eugenol and apigenin, found in basil, parsley, and rosemary, have anti-inflammatory properties that can help with conditions such as arthritis, asthma, and bowel inflammation. A cup of fresh sage and rosemary tea is wonderful for digestion or even a cough.

herby sweet oven fries

WHO NEEDS DEEP-FRIED POTATOES WHEN YOU CAN HAVE THESE SWEET POTATO OVEN FRIES? THEY GO WELL WITH ANY MAIN COURSE, OR SERVE THEM WITH DIPS, SUCH AS APRICOT SALSA (PAGE 175) OR AVOCADO CREAM (PAGE 127).

4 medium **sweet potatoes**, *scrubbed*
several **oregano** *sprigs*
several **thyme** *sprigs*
good splash of olive oil
freshly ground black pepper

Preheat the oven to 350°F. Cut the sweet potatoes lengthwise into chunky, wedge-shaped pieces. Put them in a baking dish with the herbs and olive oil. Season with pepper and toss well. Bake until tender—a skewer or sharp knife will slide through easily, about 30 minutes. Drain on paper towels and serve.

white bean mash

MY FRIEND JANET KIPLING MADE THESE FOR ME ONE WINTER'S EVENING. YOU CAN
LEAVE THE COOKED BEANS UNMASHED IF YOU PREFER, EATING THEM EITHER HOT
OR COOL AS A SALAD.

splash of olive oil
1 large **onion**, peeled and
    chopped
2–3 **rosemary** sprigs
4–6 **sage** leaves
3 heaped cups cannellini
    beans or navy **beans**
    (cooked or canned and
    drained)
2 **garlic** cloves, peeled and
    finely chopped
$^2/_3$ cup water
pinch of sea salt
freshly ground black pepper
$^1/_2$ tbsp wholegrain mustard
1 heaped tbsp chopped
    parsley

Heat the olive oil in a large saucepan. Add the
onion, along with the rosemary and sage, and
cook until softened; don't let it brown. Toss in the
beans, then add the garlic, water, salt, and pepper.
Let simmer gently for about 20 minutes. Take out
the woody rosemary stems. (I leave the herb
leaves in for color.)

Mash the bean mixture well, adding the
mustard and parsley as you do so. Serve with a
tomato salad, or as a side dish with meat or fish.

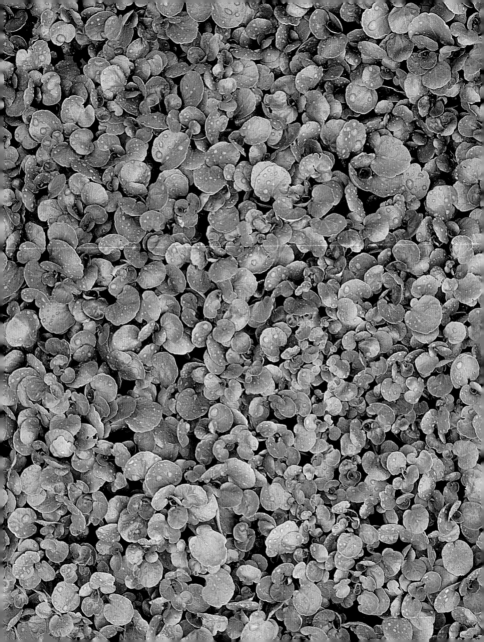

watercress

This peppery green has been eaten since ancient times and was used as a remedy for catarrh, bronchitis, and scurvy. These days, it is an underrated food, although it's packed with those all-important antioxidants, including members of the carotene family, lutein and zeaxanthin, as well as the powerful anti-inflammatory quercetin. Weight for weight, it is as rich as oranges in vitamin C, which is essential for keeping our skin regenerating well, our liver healthy, and our defences strong. With aging from oxidant damage, we're not just talking about visible external wrinkles, but also the health of our internal organs—essential for a long, healthy life. In common with other members of the cruciferous family (like broccoli and cabbage), watercress contains glucosinolates, which help the liver's detoxification capacity. One type in particular, phenylethyl isothiocyanate, has been shown to have anti-cancer properties. Watercress also helps the release of bile from the gall bladder, which is important for fat digestion, and works as a natural laxative.

monkfish with watercress sauce

YOU CAN USE ANY WHITE FISH FOR THIS DISH, BUT PEPPERY WATERCRESS
COMPLEMENTS MONKFISH PARTICULARLY WELL.

1 heaped tbsp **sunflower seeds**
1 tbsp olive oil
4 **shallots**, peeled and finely diced
1 **garlic** clove, peeled and crushed
4 portions of **monkfish** or other white **fish** fillet, each about 5 oz
juice of 1–2 **lemons**
3–4 handfuls of **watercress**, washed and roughly chopped
freshly ground black pepper
2 heaped tbsp sour cream

In a large, dry frying pan over moderate heat, toss the sunflower seeds until they are golden. Then add the olive oil and soften the shallots and garlic over low heat until they turn opaque.

Add the fish portions and cook gently for about 2 minutes, then turn and cook the other side for a couple of minutes. Sprinkle with the lemon juice, then add the watercress to the pan, stirring it around so it wilts. Season with pepper. Turn the fish again and cook until done, about 2 minutes longer; it will need around 8 minutes in total, depending on the thickness of the fillets.

Add the sour cream and heat gently, stirring it into the watercress around the fish. Serve the fish topped with the sauce.

scrambled eggs with watercress

CREAMY SOFT EGGS AND SHARP, FRESH-TASTING WATERCRESS MAKE A WONDERFUL COMBINATION. FOR A RICHER, MORE DECADENT VERSION, SERVE IT WITH SLICES OF SMOKED SALMON AND A SPRINKLING OF FRESHLY CHOPPED DILL.

6 **eggs**
freshly ground black pepper
pinch of salt
dash of milk or **soymilk**
1 tsp butter
2 handfuls of **watercress**,
    washed and roughly
    chopped
wholegrain rye toast, lightly
    buttered, for serving

Beat the eggs in a bowl with pepper, salt, and a dash of milk.

Heat the butter in a saucepan, add the eggs, and stir constantly over very low heat until they are the texture you like—the secret lies in cooking them slowly. A minute or so before they are ready, stir in the watercress so it wilts.

Serve on top of hot, lightly buttered wholegrain rye toast.

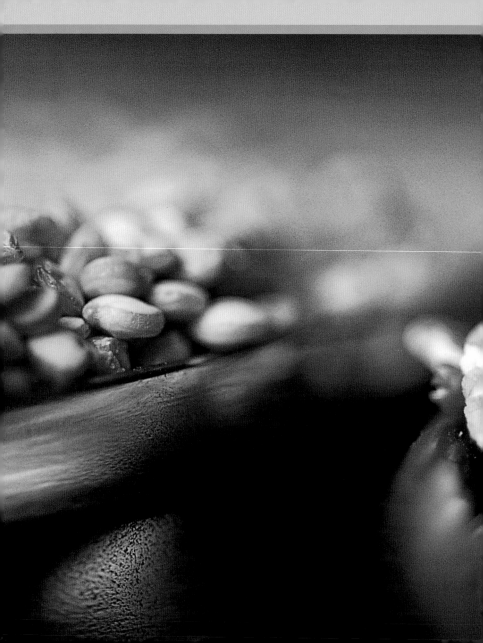

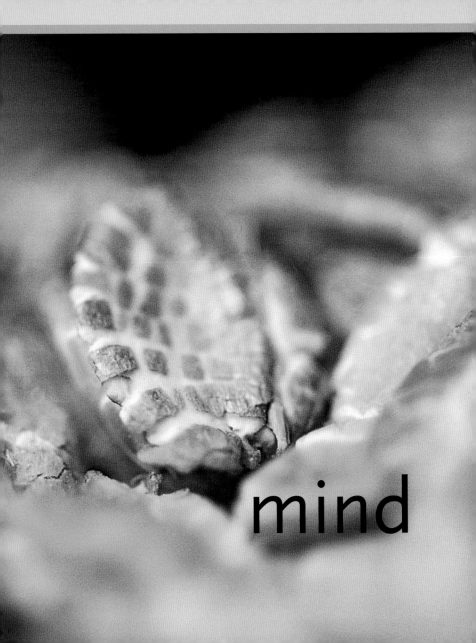

mind

The wonderfoods in this section contain nutrients that help to balance out moods, to calm you down when you are anxious, and to get a good night's sleep. Even if you are someone who relies on alcohol or drugs to help you relax, these foods can help you chill out further. Eaten as part of a varied intake, they could even help you to reduce your dependence on ultimately detrimental, short-term solutions.

Certain foods contain natural substances that help quiet down the nervous system, such as the gramine in oats. The minerals calcium and magnesium work in tandem to balance the nervous system and muscle contraction-relaxation. Both sunflower and sesame seeds are good sources of these two minerals, while yogurt provides calcium. Just working on calming the nervous system, however, is not the only answer. It's also important to support the body's stress response by keeping the adrenal glands well nourished with nutrients such as pantothenic acid, which is found in seeds and whole grains.

Keeping blood-sugar levels well balanced is an important part of reducing anxiety, restful sleep, and even moods. Having three meals a day, plus two snacks if necessary, can help this, by ensuring that the body does not go for too long without fuel. Eating a protein-rich food such as yogurt, chicken, or eggs means that the release of energy from the meal is sustained rather than sudden. These two strategies alone are a good start in reducing anxiety and low moods; they also put you in a position where you are less likely to need the lift or the downer from sugar, caffeine, cigarettes, drugs, or booze.

One of the chemicals that the body produces naturally for good moods is the neurotransmitter (nerve messenger molecule) serotonin. The amino acid tryptophan—found in chicken, yogurt, and seeds, among other foods—is one of the raw ingredients for making serotonin. Others are B vitamins and zinc, found in the same foods and in whole grains. In order for serotonin to, in effect, transmit a message from one cell to the next, the gateway to the cell—its membrane—needs to be in good shape. Healthy membranes incorporate important fats such as those derived from seeds and phosphatidylcholine, a substance derived from the choline in eggs.

There is more, of course, to keeping calm and happy than keeping your cells on good form, serotonin production, and even blood-sugar levels. If patches of stress seem to stretch on forever, assessing and dealing with what is going on in your life, your lifestyle, and the way you react to events—with professional help if need be—is fundamental.

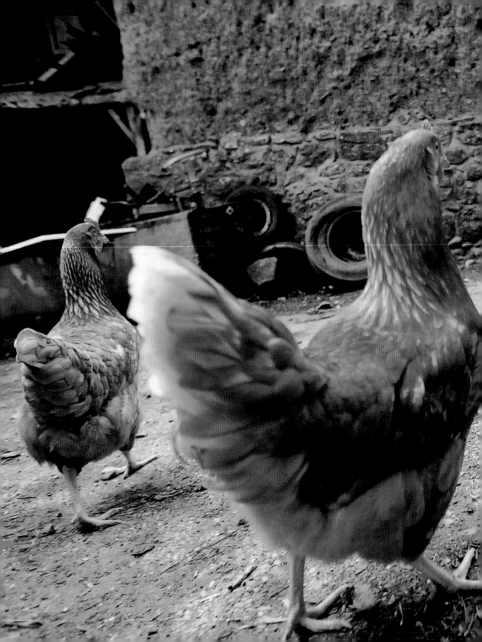

turkey & chicken

You don't need to wait for the holidays to have turkey on the table, as portions are now readily available. Skinless turkey breast is about the leanest meat there is, so it's an excellent source of protein—one portion giving you as much as half your daily need. Organic, free-range chicken is good, too, and both meats contain the amino acid tryptophan. The body can convert tryptophan into serotonin, in effect, a "happy hormone" that also helps you feel relaxed. Turkey and chicken provide doses of B vitamins—needed to make energy, to respond to stress, and also to actually turn tryptophan into serotonin. These lean meats are rich in the mineral zinc, which has countless uses in the body; studies have shown many people with depression are low in zinc. Having protein food, such as turkey or chicken, makes a meal more satisfying for longer, which in turn helps keep energy, moods, and concentration more even. The majority of chickens and turkeys are reared very intensively, so I recommend that you buy organic.

lemongrass turkey skewers

MY FRIEND, THE CHEF ALAN WICHERT, MAKES THIS WONDERFUL DISH DURING THE
HEALTHY FITNESS VACATIONS WE WORK ON TOGETHER IN MARRAKECH. IT ALWAYS
GOES DOWN WELL WITH GUESTS. IF YOU CAN'T FIND LEMONGRASS YOU CAN USE
METAL OR WOODEN SKEWERS (SOAKING THE LATTER BEFORE COOKING).

juice of 1 **lime**
juice of ½ **orange**
½ tbsp harissa paste
½ tbsp cumin seeds
½ tbsp fennel seeds
1 tbsp olive oil
2 large, skinless, boneless
   turkey breast halves
8 lemongrass stalks
1 zucchini, sliced into
   ½-inch disks
1 red **bell pepper**, cored,
   seeded, and cut into
   squares
8 shiitake **mushrooms**, cut
   in half
½ **pineapple**, peeled, cored,
   and cubed

In a large bowl, mix together the lime juice, orange juice, harissa, cumin seeds, fennel seeds, and olive oil. Cut the turkey into bite-sized chunks, add to the bowl, and toss well. Cover and let marinate in a cool place, ideally for at least 2 hours.

Thread the turkey pieces onto the lemongrass "skewers," alternating with the zucchini, red pepper, mushrooms, and pineapple. Prepare the grill fire, or preheat a ridged, castiron grill pan (oil this lightly). Cook the skewers, turning occasionally, until evenly colored and the turkey is cooked through, about 10 minutes.

Serve the skewers with Mango & pineapple salsa (page 134) and brown rice.

crusted baked chicken

A TASTY CRUST FLAVORS SKINLESS CHICKEN THIGHS AND HELPS TO KEEP THEM
MOIST DURING COOKING.

1 red **onion**, peeled and
    quartered
1 **garlic** clove, peeled
1 heaped tbsp chopped
    lemon **thyme**
1 tsp balsamic vinegar
2 heaped tbsp freshly grated
    Parmesan cheese
1 tbsp olive oil
$^1/_3$ cup **sunflower seeds**
8 **chicken** thighs, skin
    removed

Preheat the oven to 350°F. Using a mortar and
pestle, pound the onion, garlic, lemon thyme,
balsamic vinegar, Parmesan, and olive oil together.
Add the sunflower seeds and work to a rough
paste, adding a spoonful of water, if necessary.

Lay the chicken pieces in a baking dish and
smother them generously with the crust mixture.
Pour a little water into the dish, just enough to
cover the bottom, then bake until the chicken is
cooked through, about 30 minutes.

This is delicious with brown rice or buckwheat
and with Green spice stir-fry (page 95) or steamed
broccoli florets.

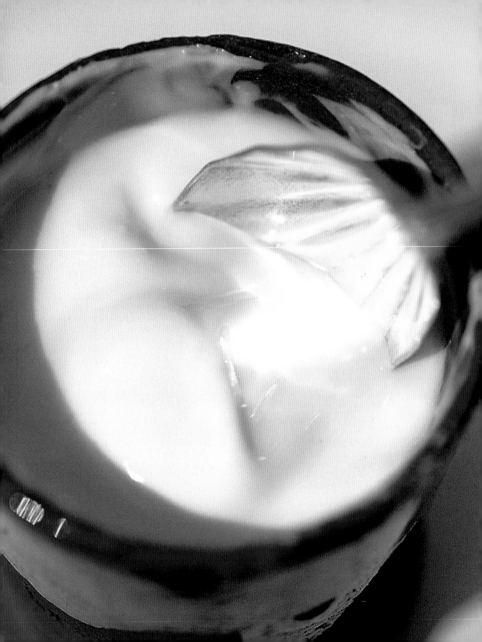

yogurt

Ever since cows were first domesticated, humans have been eating fermented milk, and its benefits have long been recognized. Yogurt is made by adding lactobacillus and bifidobacteria cultures to milk, but it's important to buy "live" yogurts as some are pasteurized after the culture is added, killing it off. Live bacteria are well-known beneficial inhabitants of our digestive tracts as they help maintain the correct acidity, enhance immunity, and aid digestion. Lactobacillus and bifidobacteria have also been shown to help lower cholesterol levels. Yogurt is a good protein food, particularly for vegetarians. It contains tryptophan, the precursor of serotonin, the mood-booster. Some people who react badly to milk products are fine with yogurt, because bacteria ferment it by eating the milk sugar (lactose), making it more digestible. Like all milk products, yogurt is a rich source of calcium, which is essential for healthy bones but also for muscles to work properly, and for nerves to fire their messages efficiently.

salmon with seaweed sauce

ALTHOUGH I'VE USED SALMON HERE, YOU CAN COOK ANY FISH YOU FANCY TO GO
WITH THIS SAUCE.

½ cup plain **yogurt**
½-inch piece fresh **ginger**,
    peeled and grated
1 **garlic** clove, peeled and
    grated
grated zest and juice of
    1 **lime**
2 tbsp toasted **sesame** oil
½ tsp cayenne pepper
4 **salmon** (or other **fish**)
    steaks, each about 6 oz
2 heaped tbsp dried
    seaweed, such as arame
    or hijiki

Mix the yogurt, ginger, garlic, lime zest and juice,
sesame oil, and cayenne together in a shallow
bowl. Add the fish and swish it around in the
mixture to coat it well. Set aside to marinate for
about 20 minutes.

Meanwhile, put the seaweed in a mug and
pour in just enough boiling water to cover it. Let
steep for 4–5 minutes.

Put the salmon steaks and marinade in a large
frying pan over moderate heat, along with the
seaweed and its water. Lower the heat when the
liquid start to bubble and cook until the fish
steaks are done, 10–15 minutes, turning them
halfway through.

Accompany with steamed or stir-fried kale and
brown rice.

berry fool

THIS DESSERT IS SO HEALTHY THAT YOU CAN GET AWAY WITH HAVING A BUTTERY, CRUMBLY SHORTBREAD COOKIE TO ACCOMPANY IT! USE THICK YOGURT SO THE FOOL WON'T BE TOO RUNNY. WHEN FRESH BERRIES AREN'T IN SEASON IT'S FINE TO USE FROZEN ONES.

1 lb mixed **berries**, such as raspberries, blueberries, and strawberries
1 cup thick plain **yogurt** (ideally Greek-style)
1 tbsp sugar or alternative equivalent (see page 10)

Put the ingredients into a blender, saving a few whole berries for serving, and whiz until evenly blended. Divide among individual dishes and top each serving with a couple of berries.

Serve shortbread cookies or small meringues alongside.

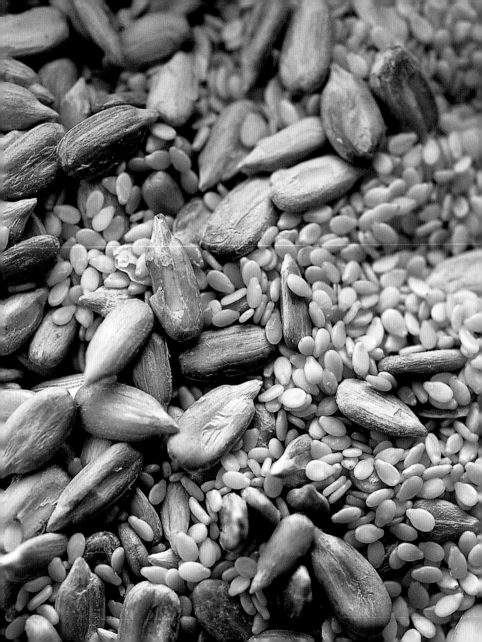

sunflower seeds & sesame seeds

Both sunflower seeds, from the studded centers of the vivid yellow flowers, and tiny sesame seeds, which in ancient India were a symbol of immortality, are powerhouses of nutrients. Both seeds are good sources of vitamin E, plus omega-6 and monounsaturated fats, all of which help minimize heart disease as well as boost the elasticity of skin. They are also rich in calcium and magnesium, needed for relaxation and contraction of muscles (including the heart) and bone health. Magnesium is required for each cell to produce energy, yet it is also considered the "calming" mineral. The zinc and selenium in sunflower and sesame seeds (as well sesamol and other chemicals) are important antioxidants. Low levels of zinc are associated with poor immunity, infertility, bad skin, and pantothenic acid in the seeds is essential for a healthy response to stress. Sesame seeds, because of their size, are often left undigested, which means that the nutrient content is missed. When chewed thoroughly, though, or used as a paste (tahini), you can get their full benefits.

sunny salad

EVEN IF YOU CAN'T GET HOLD OF ANY OF THE FLOWERS FOR THIS, IT'S STILL A COLORFUL SALAD, BRIMMING WITH GOODNESS. IF YOU'VE NEVER TASTED COLD-PRESSED SUNFLOWER OIL BEFORE, YOU'LL BE KNOCKED OUT BY ITS GORGEOUSLY NUTTY, RICH FLAVOR. BORAGE IS KNOWN AS A CALMING HERB.

*1 yellow **bell pepper**, cored, seeded, and chopped*
*handful of **watercress** leaves*
1/2 red-leaved lettuce, such as lollo rosso
selection of nasturtium, borage, and marigold flowers
*2 **scallions**, trimmed and sliced*
*1 heaped tbsp **sunflower seeds***
*1 tbsp cold-pressed **sunflower oil***
capful of cider vinegar

Toss all the ingredients together just before serving, as a side salad with a main dish such as Sesame-studded mackerel (opposite).

sesame-studded mackerel

I OFTEN COOK MACKEREL THIS WAY, BUT YOU CAN USE ANY FISH YOU LIKE.

$^1/_3$ cup **sesame seeds**

2 heaped tbsp chopped chives

4 **mackerel** fillets

a little toasted **sesame** oil

1 **lime**, cut into wedges, for serving

Mix the sesame seeds and chives together on a large plate, then press both sides of the fish fillets onto them, so that the seeds as well as the chives adhere.

Heat a ridged, castiron grill pan or frying pan and add a little sesame oil. Cook the fish for 2–3 minutes each side, depending on the thickness of the fillets.

Serve with lime wedges and accompany with soba noodles and a salad or stir-fried spinach.

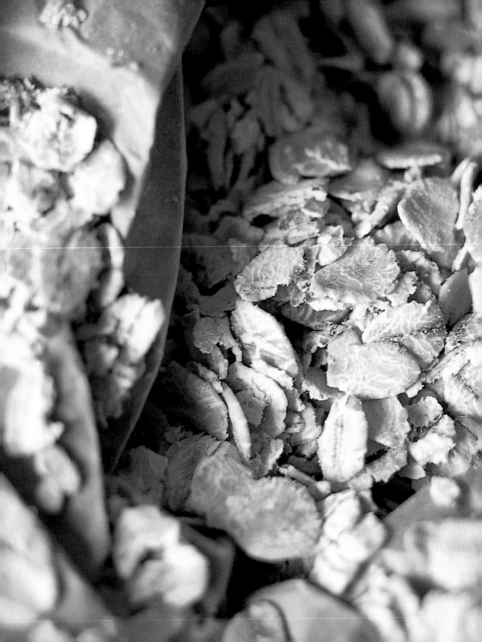

oats

Good, old-fashioned oats are a remarkably versatile grain with wide-ranging health properties. In addition to being a good source of carbohydrates, they are high in both soluble and insoluble fiber. This means they are digested slowly and don't raise blood-sugar levels dramatically. Consequently, oats will keep both mood and energy levels even for a while after they are eaten—making them an ideal breakfast food. The fiber contributes to a healthy gut, not just keeping you regular, but also binding to waste products. Studies have shown that oats can also help lower cholesterol. Herbalists recommend oat extracts to help calm anxiety and depression, which is probably why oat tincture has been recommended for people trying to quit smoking. Oats are loaded with B vitamins, vitamin E, and important minerals such as iron and zinc. All of these are needed for a healthy nervous system, as well as much, much more. Oats are also one of the richest food sources of silicon, needed for healthy skin and bones. Use this versatile grain to make oatmeal, oaty snack bars, or crisp toppings.

crunchy plum crisp

THIS A WONDERFUL VERSION OF THE TRADITIONAL DESSERT. YOU CAN REPLACE
THE PLUMS WITH APPLES, RHUBARB, OR BERRIES, IF PREFERRED.

3 cups **muesli**
1 tsp ground **cinnamon**
2 heaped tbsp **pumpkin seeds**
10 **walnuts**, shelled and broken into pieces
3 tbsp butter, in pieces
1³/₄ lb **plums**, halved and pitted
4–5 star anise
1 heaped tbsp brown sugar
¹/₃ cup water
FOR SERVING
²/₃ cup plain **yogurt**
¹/₂ tsp vanilla extract, or to taste

Preheat the oven to 350°F. Combine the muesli, cinnamon, pumpkin seeds, and walnuts in a large mixing bowl. Add the butter and rub in using your fingertips until there are no lumps of butter left. Alternatively, you can melt the butter and mix it in that way.

Lay the plums and star anise in a baking dish and sprinkle with the sugar and water. Spoon the muesli mixture over the top of the plums, so that they are well covered. Bake until the plums are soft when tested with a skewer, about 40 minutes.

Mix the yogurt with the vanilla extract to serve alongside, or, more indulgently, have vanilla ice cream or custard sauce.

fruity oatmeal

THERE'S NO BETTER START TO THE DAY THAN A BOWL OF HOT OATMEAL. ADDING
FRUIT GIVES AN UNUSUAL TEXTURE AND SWEETNESS, ALTHOUGH IT CAN BE ADDED
AFTER YOU'VE COOKED THE OATMEAL, IF YOU PREFER. YOU COULD REPLACE THE
APPLE OR PEAR WITH 2–3 TBSP STEWED RHUBARB OR A FEW STEWED PLUMS.
SERVES 2

½ cup quick-cooking
    rolled **oats**
about 1 cup milk or **soymilk**
1 **apple** or **pear**, grated
1 tsp **honey** or maple syrup
2 heaped tbsp **High five
    mix** (page 154)

Put the oats in a saucepan, add water to cover,
and stir with a wooden spoon over low heat. As
the oats begin to absorb the water, slowly start to
add the milk, stirring all the time. Add the fruit.
Each time the oatmeal starts to thicken, add a
little more milk to keep it slightly runny.

When the oats are cooked—this should take
about 5 minutes—stir in the honey or maple
syrup, top with the High five mix, and serve.

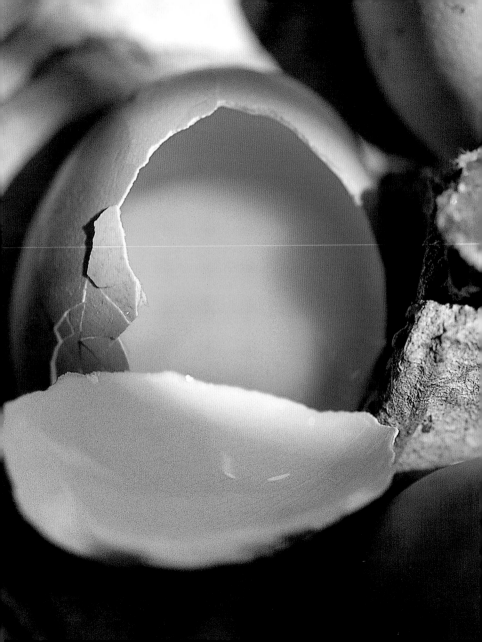

egg

Eggs get a bad press due to their cholesterol content, but as an excellent source of protein, vitamins, minerals, and, most interestingly, unsaturated fats, they are a wonderfood in a neat shell. Of the 5 grams of fat in an egg, most is monounsaturated (like olive oil), which actually helps lower the risk of heart disease. Anyway, we need some cholesterol for a healthy brain and for making the sex and stress hormones. Egg yolk is the richest known source of choline, which helps keep cholesterol fluid, preventing it from clogging up arteries. Choline also makes up cell membranes, helps the body process fats, and converts to acetylcholine, an important memory molecule in the brain. The yolk's rich color comes from beneficial antioxidants, lutein and zeaxanthin. Eggs are a great source of iron, zinc, and selenium, plus A and B vitamins. The truth is an egg is as healthy as the chicken that laid it—so buy only organic or free-range and an egg a day could help keep the doctor away.

asparagus & sunchoke tortilla

IF YOU CAN'T GET HOLD OF JERUSALEM ARTICHOKES, USE BABY NEW POTATOES
FOR THIS SPANISH-STYLE OMELET. YOU'LL NEED A FRYING PAN THAT'S SUITABLE
TO USE BRIEFLY UNDER THE BROILER.

8 *Jerusalem artichokes*,
   scrubbed
juice of ¹/₂ **lemon**
8 **eggs**
4–6 **basil** *leaves, torn*
freshly ground black pepper
pinch of fine sea salt
splash of olive oil
handful of **spinach** *leaves,*
   roughly chopped
8 *thin* **asparagus** *spears,*
   cut into pieces
2 *medium* **tomatoes**, *sliced*

Cook the Jerusalem artichokes in boiling water to cover, with the lemon juice, until they feel tender when pierced with a skewer, about 15 minutes. Drain and let cool, then slice thickly.

Beat the eggs with the basil and seasoning. Preheat the broiler.

Heat the olive oil in a large frying pan and add the egg mixture. Scatter the spinach, asparagus, artichokes, and tomatoes evenly over the egg. Cook the tortilla for about 3 minutes (don't stir it), then place it under the broiler to cook for a minute or two until it's golden brown all over.

Serve the tortilla cut into wedges, with a Wonderfoods green salad (page 111).

broccoli-polenta quiche

POLENTA FORMS THE BASE FOR THIS "QUICHE," RATHER THAN THE USUAL PASTRY.
YOU COULD USE PRETTY MUCH ANY CHEESE YOU HAVE IN THE REFRIGERATOR.

2 cups vegetable or chicken
    stock
1¼ cups cornmeal
2 heaped tbsp freshly grated
    Parmesan cheese
walnut-sized piece of butter
a little olive oil
3 **eggs**
1 cup milk
½ tsp mustard powder
½ tsp freshly grated nutmeg
freshly ground black pepper
pinch of fine sea salt
3 **scallions**, trimmed and
    finely sliced
4 oz **broccoli**, cut into very
    small florets
½ cup shredded Gruyère or
    strong Cheddar cheese

Preheat the oven to 350°F. Bring the stock to a boil in a large saucepan. Turn down the heat and slowly add the cornmeal, whisking constantly to avoid it becoming lumpy. Add the Parmesan and butter as you continue to whisk. Cook, stirring regularly, until the polenta is very thick and comes away from the sides of the pan easily, about 10 minutes.

Smear the bottom of a 9-inch tart pan with olive oil, pour in the polenta, and bake for 30 minutes.

Meanwhile, in a bowl, beat the eggs, milk, mustard, nutmeg, pepper, and salt together. Scatter the scallions, broccoli florets, and half of the Gruyère evenly over the polenta base. Carefully pour the egg mixture over and sprinkle with the rest of the cheese. Bake until the filling is set, about 30 minutes.

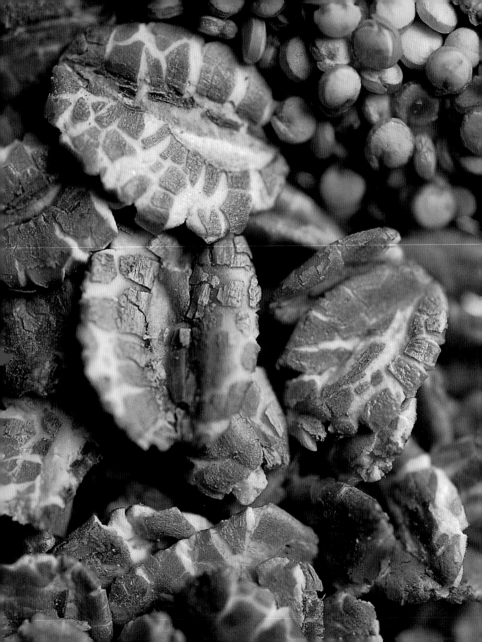

quinoa & rye

When the Spanish conquered Latin America, they forbade the cultivation of quinoa, realizing what a fortifying, revered food it was. Pronounced *keen-wa* in its native land, it is known as the "mother grain," indicating its significance—nutritionally and spiritually. When cooked, part of it separates, giving each grain a small halo! Quinoa contains significantly more protein than other grain foods and has the full range of essential amino acids. It also provides a spectrum of B vitamins, including pantothenic acid (B5), which is essential for the adrenal glands to mount a healthy stress response. Probably because of its hardy nature, rye is most popular in the coldest parts of the world. It is particularly high in non-cellulose polysaccharides (fiber), which bind well with water, leaving you feeling more satisfied for longer after eating. It's also helpful for those managing their blood-sugar balance, including diabetics. Rye is rich in antioxidants called phenolics and plant lignans, which protect the body from cancer and heart disease, and can help reduce the uncomfortable symptoms linked to the menopause.

fish stew with quinoa

THIS IS A VERY LIGHT, BROTHY STEW WITH A SUBTLE BLEND OF FLAVORS. YOU CAN USE ANY SEAFOOD YOU FANCY, THOUGH FIRM-TEXTURED WHITE FISH AND A MIX OF SHELLFISH—SHRIMP, MUSSELS, CLAMS, ETC.—WORKS BEST.

a little olive oil
*1 small **onion**, peeled and finely diced*
*3 **garlic** cloves, peeled and crushed*
1/2 tsp cayenne pepper
*1/2 tsp ground **turmeric***
1/2 tsp smoked paprika
*1 green **bell pepper**, cored, seeded, and chopped*
*4 medium **tomatoes**, peeled and chopped*
2 tbsp capers
generous splash of white wine
1 1/4 cups vegetable or fish stock
*7 oz filleted **fish**, such as monkfish or chunky cod*
about 8 large, raw shrimp, peeled and deveined
about 8 mussels, cleaned
*2 heaped tbsp chopped **parsley***

FOR THE QUINOA
*1 1/4 cups **quinoa***
2 1/2 cups water

Heat the olive oil in a large pan and soften the onion and garlic with the spices over low heat. Then add the green pepper, tomatoes, and capers and stir for 2 or 3 minutes. Pour in the wine and stock and bring to a boil, then cover and let simmer for about 20 minutes, stirring occasionally.

Meanwhile, cook the quinoa. Rinse it well, then put it into a pan with the water and bring to a boil. Cover, turn down the heat to a simmer, and cook for about 15 minutes.

Cut the fish into bite-sized chunks and add them to the tomato broth. Cover and cook for about 2 minutes, then add the shrimp and mussels. Continue to cook until the shrimp turn pink and the mussels open. Serve sprinkled with the chopped parsley, on a pile of quinoa.

designer muesli

THIS MUESLI TAKES SECONDS TO MAKE, ALL TO YOUR OWN SPECIFICATIONS. GOOD
HEALTHFOOD STORES AND WHOLEFOOD MARKETS SELL A RANGE OF OTHER GRAINS
THAT YOU CAN ADD TO THE MIX. AND, OF COURSE, YOU CAN ADD ANY OTHER
NUTS, SEEDS, OR DRIED FRUITS YOU LIKE. SOME GRAINS, SUCH AS QUINOA, ARE
BEST PUFFED, AS THEY ARE INEDIBLE RAW. *MAKES 12–15 SERVINGS*

*2 cups **rye** flakes*
*2 cups **oat** flakes*
2 cups barley flakes
*2 cups puffed **quinoa***
*2 heaped tbsp **sunflower
seeds***
*2 heaped tbsp **pumpkin
seeds***
3 heaped tbsp raisins
*8 dried **apricots**, finely
chopped*
FOR SERVING
*milk, plain **yogurt**, or
soymilk*

Mix all the ingredients together in a large storage
container. Serve yourself a bowlful with fresh milk,
plain yogurt, or soymilk. Top with fresh fruit,
if desired.

NOTE If you have a sensitive digestion, soak your
bowl of muesli overnight in milk or apple juice.

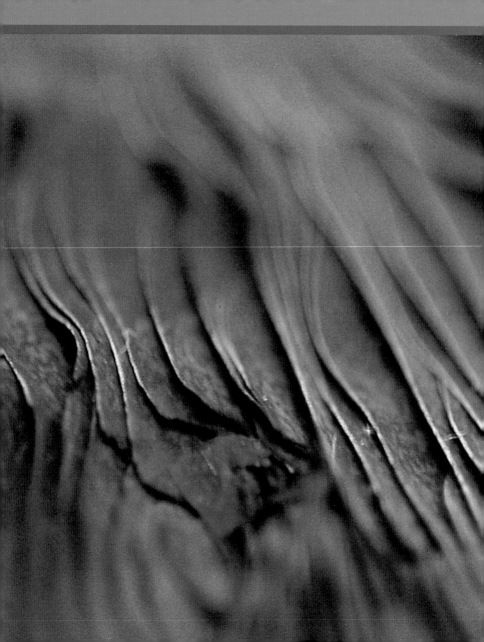

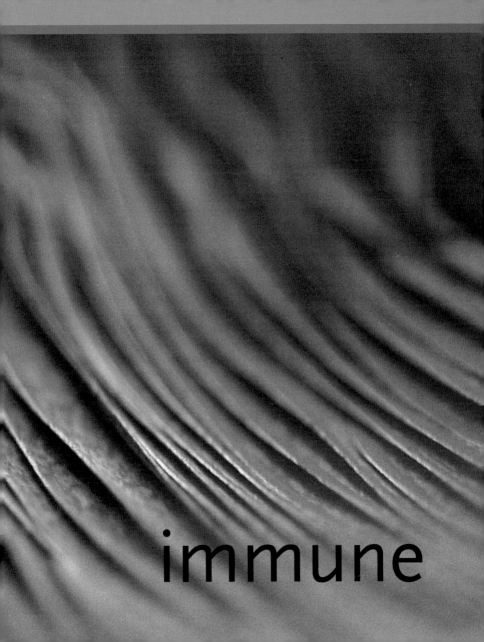

immune

Old-fashioned remedies are often still used, because they've withstood the test of time, and now scientists are showing that they make good modern sense, too. Lemons for a cold, onions for a cough, shiitake mushrooms to ward off flu—these are just some of the immunity-boosters you might find in an old wives' book of wonderfoods, and in mine too. However, having tried it, I can't say that I would recommend homemade onion syrup, even if it did do the trick! The foods featured in this section of Wonderfoods are packed with vitamins, minerals, and other naturally occurring substances that help strengthen our body's defences in the face of infection.

Our immune systems are remarkably intricate, consisting of countless sites and substances around the body that deal with potential pathogens—harmful, tiny organisms such as viruses, bacteria, and fungi. Not only are there special defence chemicals in our skin and tears, but also all passages that open externally, such as our lungs and digestive tract, are lined with countless immune soldiers to neutralize would-be pathogens. If invaders manage to get through the first line of defences, further trouble lies in store for them in the form of immune cells that either patrol the body or sit waiting to pounce on anything that comes along. The body also produces special immune cells and substances to combat specific invaders; others detect and clear up suspect cells such as cancerous ones.

Not surprisingly, each person's immune system reacts at least slightly differently owing to our different genes and environments, even when we are exposed to the same pathogen. In some cases, one person may not get sick at all, while another succumbs completely to the same cold virus or stomach bug to which both were exposed. What makes the difference? The terrain into which the bug lands. Keep your body well up on nutrients that the immune system needs, such as those in these wonderfoods, and you'll be less likely to get ill. And if you do, you'll probably recover much more rapidly.

A good dose of immune wonderfoods is not all you'll need for keeping illness at bay. Stress is a big enemy of the immune system, as is too little sleep, not to mention the obvious factors like smoking and a high intake of alcohol. If, though, you have a diet that is high in immune wonderfoods, yet you still fall prey to infections regularly, you should work with a professional to see what could be pulling the rug out from underneath your body's defences.

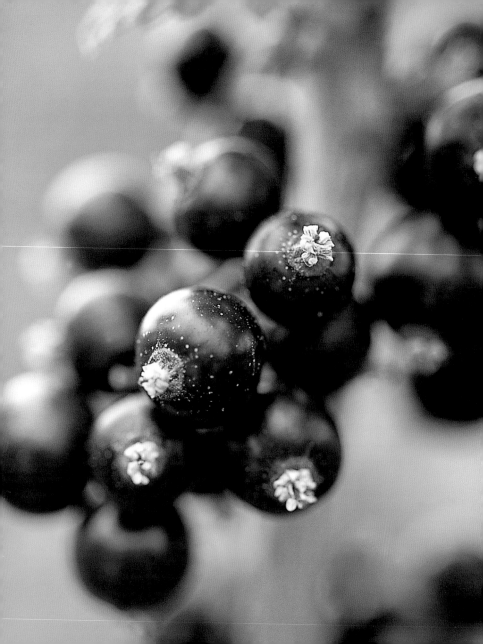

black currants

Historically, black currants were grown for their medicinal properties and for turning into wine, or for making hot drinks to ease a sore throat. Because they are relatively tart, they are rarely eaten alone, and these days, the closest many people get to them is in a sweetened syrup that shouts about its rich vitamin C content. Indeed, black currants contain three times as much of this vital vitamin as oranges, weight for weight. Forget the syrup though, with its high sugar content, and eat the fruit with other foods that compensate for the sharpness. Black currants are not just an extraordinary source of vitamin C, but also of its companion antioxidants, bioflavonoids, which are well known for boosting the body's defences. These compounds also help the condition of blood vessels, the skin, and the stress response. In addition, the fiber and seeds in black currants have long made them a good remedy for constipation, as they encourage the bowels to work smoothly.

black-currant smoothie

I LOVE THE CONTRAST OF SWEET, THICK BANANA AND TANGY BLACK CURRANTS IN THIS REFRESHING DRINK. YOU CAN MAKE IT THROUGHOUT THE WINTER USING BLACK CURRANTS CANNED IN NATURAL JUICE. CRUNCH WELL ON THE BLACK-CURRANT SEEDS, AS THEY ARE FULL OF HEALTHY ESSENTIAL FATTY ACIDS. *SERVES 2*

1 **banana**

2 heaped tbsp **black currants**

$1/3$ cup plain **yogurt**

1 cup **apple** juice (or the juice from the black currants, if using canned ones)

Whiz everything up in a blender, pour into glasses, and drink immediately.

NOTE This is enough for two large glasses.

black currant & apricot slice

THIS SLICE IS RELATIVELY IMPRESSIVE FOR THE EFFORT REQUIRED TO MAKE IT AND IT'S DELICIOUS EATEN WARM, WITH VANILLA ICE CREAM. YOU COULD MAKE INDIVIDUAL SQUARE OR TRIANGULAR PASTRIES, IF YOU PREFER.

*7 oz puff pastry, thawed
  if frozen*
*1/4 cup ground **almonds***
*3 tbsp roughly chopped
  almonds*
1/2 tbsp butter, softened
*3 tsp **walnut** or **hemp** oil*
1/2 tsp vanilla extract
*1 tbsp **honey***
*1/3 cup **black currants***
*4 **apricots**, halved, pitted
  and sliced*

Preheat the oven to 400°F. Line a baking sheet with parchment paper. Cut a rectangle of pastry 10–12 inches long and 4–5 inches wide and lay it on the paper.

In a bowl, mix the ground and chopped almonds, butter, 2 tsp oil, the vanilla, and honey. Spread this mix over the pastry, leaving a 1/2-inch margin all around. Lay the black currants and apricots on top of the almond mixture. Brush the pastry edges with the remaining oil.

Bake until the pastry edges are puffed up and golden, about 15 minutes. Eat warm.

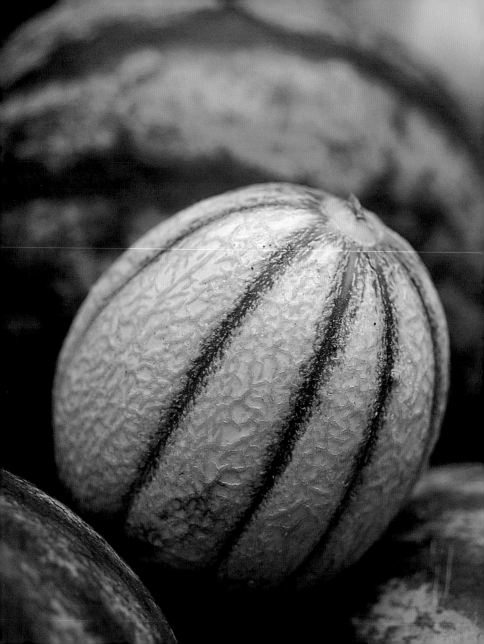

watermelon &
melon

Apart from the refreshing juiciness, the crunchy texture, and the taste, watermelon has a lot to offer your health. For thousands of years, watermelons have been valued in Africa and Asia (where aridity and polluted water are common) for their high content of sweet water. An impressive 90% of the flesh is water, so it is a refreshing cleanser and a diuretic. The red flesh is rich in powerful antioxidant nutrients, such as water-soluble vitamin C and fat-soluble lycopene and beta-carotene—all important for helping your body's detoxification, fighting infections, protecting the eyes and lungs, slowing down aging and countering inflammation. The seeds are loaded with yet more antioxidants, such as zinc, selenium, and vitamin E, plus essential fats, so crunch them to get the full benefit. Pretty much all these nutrients contribute to fertility and sexual performance. Like watermelons, although not strictly related, melons are loaded with water and, particularly cantaloupe, with beta-carotene.

watermelon & watercress salad

THIS HAS TO BE ONE OF THE MOST ZINGY, REFRESHING SALADS POSSIBLE, BUT, TO MAKE IT MORE SO, YOU COULD ADD SOME GRAPEFRUIT SEGMENTS.

*2 large slices of **watermelon***
*2 large handfuls of **watercress**, trimmed*
*½ red **onion**, peeled and very finely sliced*
*½-inch piece fresh **ginger**, peeled and grated*
2 tsp tamari or soy sauce
*juice of 1 **lime***
*4–6 **Brazil nuts**, roughly chopped*
1 heaped tbsp chopped cilantro leaves

Cut the watermelon flesh away from the skin and chop the flesh into bite-sized pieces. Roughly chop the watercress and put it into a bowl with the watermelon and red onion.

Mix the ginger, tamari, and lime juice together in a small bowl. Pour over the salad, add the nuts and cilantro, and toss to mix. Serve at once.

retro melon cocktail

BLENDING THE ENTIRE WATERMELON—SEEDS AND ALL—MEANS THAT YOU GET THE MAXIMUM NUTRIENT VALUE, AS WELL AS GREAT TASTE AND TEXTURE. THIS IS GOOD FOR HANGOVERS, OR ADD A SHOT OF VODKA TO EACH GLASS.

$^{1}/_{2}$ **melon**, *such as cantaloupe*
4 *large chunks of* **watermelon**, *skin removed*
3–4 *mint leaves*

Using a melon baller or teaspoon, scoop small balls from the cantaloupe and set aside.

Put the watermelon flesh and seeds in a blender with the mint and whiz until smooth. Pour the watermelon smoothie into tall glasses. Push the melon balls onto toothpicks, balance on the edge of the glasses, and serve.

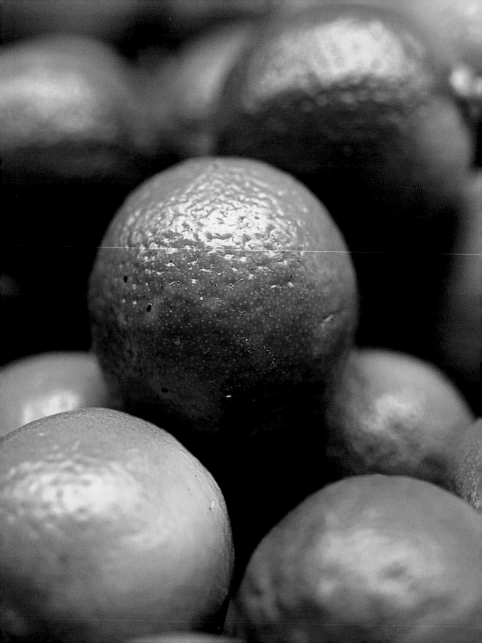

citrus fruit

As is so often the case with old wives' tales, there is more than a grain of truth that orange juice or a hot lemon drink will help you fight off a cold. Famously packed with the antioxidant vitamin C, citrus fruits give a good boost to the immune system. Vitamin C enhances the activity of white blood cells, increases the response of interferon (against viruses), and promotes antibodies. But there's a lot more to citrus fruits than that. The vitamin C is also important for the liver to work efficiently, and for healthy skin. The bitterness along with the limonene in lemons and limes stimulate the gall bladder, which helps the liver and digestion. Citrus fruits also contain bioflavonoids, such as rutin and quercitrin. These powerful antioxidants, in tandem with vitamin C, are particularly important for the health of blood vessels, so they have an impact on the cardiovascular system and help deter varicose veins. Compounds in citrus peel called polymethoxylated flavones have cholesterol-lowering effects.

tangy citrus couscous

THIS MAKES A GOOD SUMMER SALAD FOR A PICNIC OR BARBECUE AND GOES WELL
WITH GRILLED FISH OR SHRIMP.

1 heaped cup couscous
*1³/4 cups freshly squeezed
mixed **grapefruit** and
orange juice*
*1 red **bell pepper**, cored,
seeded, and chopped*
*1 zucchini, trimmed and
finely sliced*
*2 **scallions**, trimmed and
finely sliced*
*1 **garlic** clove, peeled
and crushed*
*2 heaped tbsp finely
chopped mint*
*2 heaped tbsp chopped
cilantro*
2 tbsp olive oil
24 black olives

Put the couscous in a bowl and pour on the fruit
juice. Let the couscous sit for about an hour,
forking it through occasionally.

Prepare the other ingredients in the meantime.
When the couscous is soft, add all the other
ingredients, toss to mix everything together well,
and serve immediately.

shrimp with lime-chile sauce

YOU COULD USE THIS MARINADE WITH ANY CHUNKY FISH OR SCALLOPS—TRY A MIXTURE OF SEAFOOD WITH SHRIMP THREADED ONTO THE SKEWERS.

1 heaped tsp cumin seeds
grated zest and juice of
*   1 lime*
1 garlic clove, peeled
*   and crushed*
1 tbsp sweet chile sauce
12 large raw shrimp, peeled,
*   but with head and last*
*   tail section left on, and*
*   deveined*

In a small, dry frying pan, toast the cumin seeds over moderate heat until they are smoking slightly and giving off an aroma. Tip them into a bowl.

Add the lime zest and juice, the garlic, and chile sauce, stirring well. Add the shrimp and swish them around in the mixture for a few minutes.

Prepare a grill fire, or preheat the broiler or a ridged, castiron grill pan (oiling it lightly). Cook the shrimp quickly for a few minutes, turning them once or twice, until they just turn pink. Eat them immediately. Tangy citrus couscous (opposite) is an ideal accompaniment.

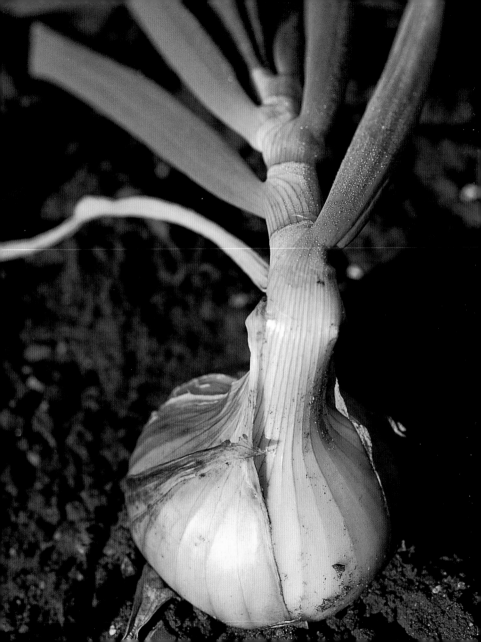

onion

I can't imagine cooking without onions, but in spiritual centers in India, they are forbidden for their ability to light your inner fire. Arousal aside, onions are widely eaten all over the world and have been used for centuries for their medicinal properties. They contain allicin and other powerful, natural antibiotics that help fight off infections, including ones in the gut caused by parasites like worms. Allicin and another chemical, allylpropyldisulfide, help lower blood sugar. Onions also contain chemicals that relax the lung muscles and help the softening of mucus, so they are good for calming a cough. For the cardiovascular system, onions act as a diuretic, help to regulate blood pressure, and help to prevent blood cells clumping. The sulfur in onions is a powerful detoxifier that boosts the liver, cleanses the gut, helps clear out toxic metals from the body (such as lead), and makes for a healthy skin. Onions also contain the antioxidant quercetin, which calms inflammation in the lungs (such as with asthma), helps protect against cancer, and strengthens blood vessels.

sweet red onion polenta

THIS IS INSPIRED BY PISSALADIÈRE, A CARAMELIZED ONION PIZZA FROM THE SOUTH OF FRANCE. YOU CAN LEAVE OUT THE ANCHOVIES IF YOU'RE VEGETARIAN OR NOT A FAN.

2 cups vegetable or chicken stock
1¼ cups cornmeal
2 tbsp freshly grated Parmesan cheese
1 tbsp butter
1 tbsp olive oil, plus extra for brushing
3 red **onions**, peeled and finely sliced
1 heaped tsp brown sugar or **honey**
8 anchovies
15–20 black olives

Preheat the oven to 350°F. Bring the stock to a boil in a large saucepan. Turn down the heat and slowly add the cornmeal, whisking constantly to avoid it becoming lumpy. Add the Parmesan and half of the butter as you continue to whisk. Cook, stirring regularly, until the polenta is very thick and comes away from the sides of the pan easily, about 10 minutes.

Rub the bottom of a 9-inch tart pan with olive oil, pour in the polenta, and bake it for 30 minutes.

Meanwhile, in a large frying pan, soften the onions in the olive oil and remaining butter with the sugar over very low heat. This always takes longer than you think—around 20 minutes. Add a little bit of water if the onions get too dry.

When the onions are soft, spread them over the polenta and top with the anchovies and olives. Eat immediately or, if preparing ahead, reheat in the oven just before serving.

dahl

MARIA PEREIRA, FROM GOA, INTRODUCED MY YOUNG TASTEBUDS TO THE
AROMATIC FLAVORS OF INDIAN COOKING AND SHOWED ME HOW TO MAKE THIS
RECIPE. DAHL JUST MEANS "LENTILS," SO IT'S ONE OF DOZENS OF RECIPES USING
THIS STAPLE. IF YOU LIKE DAHL HOT AS WELL AS SPICY, ADD A SHAKE OF HOT
CHILE POWDER TO TASTE WITH THE OTHER SPICES.

1¼ cups orange split **lentils**
1 large **onion**, peeled and
    chopped
5 **garlic** cloves
1 tsp olive oil
1 heaped tsp ground
    coriander
1 heaped tsp ground cumin
1 heaped tsp ground
    turmeric
3⅔ cups water
1 can (14 oz) crushed
    tomatoes

Wash the lentils well in a strainer and check for
any grit lurking among them. In a large saucepan,
soften the onion and garlic in the olive oil with the
spices over low heat. Don't let the onion brown—
if necessary, add a little water.

Add the lentils, water, and tomatoes and bring
to a boil. Lower the heat and let it simmer for
about an hour, stirring regularly to make sure the
dahl is not sticking. If it starts to become too
thick, add a little more water.

Eat with brown basmati rice and steamed
broccoli or spinach.

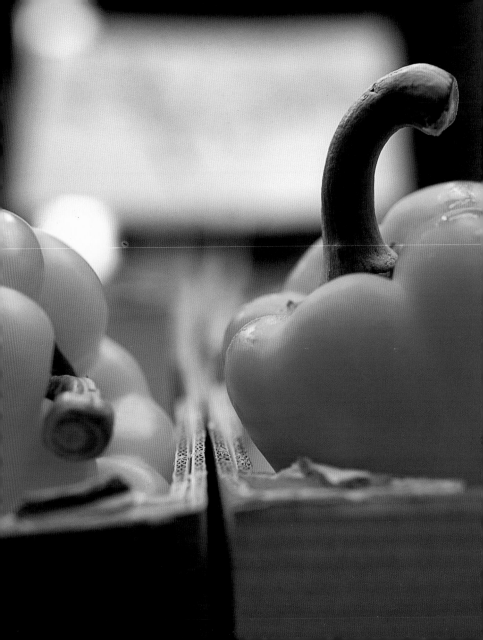

sweet pepper

The sweet pepper—of which the bell pepper is the best known variety—is a very versatile vegetable that can be eaten raw, in casseroles, roasted, stuffed, and stir-fried. Its hot cousins, chiles, have similar health benefits, if you can stand the heat. Capsaicin, the substance in peppers that determines their hotness, has antibacterial and anti-inflammatory powers, and is a natural stimulant. In force, it is great for clearing the sinuses. Even in sweet peppers, the stimulation from capsaicin boosts the circulation and digestion. Peppers are also loaded with the powerful immune-boosting vitamins A and C, so they are good for fighting off infections or keeping them at bay in the first place. These vitamins are also needed for healthy skin and lungs, and cancer protection, although much of the vitamin C in peppers is lost when they are cooked. Despite all their goodness, as a member of the nightshade family, sweet peppers may exacerbate symptoms in those with arthritis and they can irritate the gut if there is a sensitivity problem.

seared tuna & peppers

QUICK, FRESH, SIMPLE, DELICIOUS...AND GOOD FOR YOU.

4 fresh **tuna** steaks
2 **scallions**, trimmed and
    very finely sliced
1 tbsp **lemon** juice
10–12 **basil** leaves, chopped
freshly ground black pepper
1 red **bell pepper**
1 yellow **bell pepper**
a little olive oil
lemon wedges for serving

Put the tuna steaks in a dish or bowl with the scallions, lemon juice, chopped basil, and some black pepper.

Halve the peppers and remove the core and seeds, then slice lengthwise. Heat a ridged, castiron grill pan and add a little olive oil. Add the peppers and cook, turning them regularly, for about 8 minutes.

Move the peppers to one side and add the tuna to the pan. Sprinkle with the marinade and sear it to your taste—a minute or so on each side, or longer if you want it cooked through.

Serve with lemon wedges, Tangy citrus couscous (page 246), and a Wonderfoods green salad (page 111).

roasted red pepper purée

THIS SAUCE CAN BE EATEN WITH GRILLED OR SEARED FISH, CHICKEN, OR LEAN MEAT. IT CAN EVEN BE TURNED INTO A SOUP BY ADDING SOME STOCK (SEE BELOW).

8 red **bell peppers**
4 **garlic** cloves (unpeeled)
1 **onion**, cut into eighths
    (unpeeled)
splash of olive oil
2 tsp ground coriander
few **thyme** sprigs
juice of ½ **lemon**

Preheat the oven to 350°F. Toss the whole peppers, garlic, and onion in a roasting pan with a splash of olive oil, the ground coriander, and thyme. Roast until the peppers are soft, about 30 minutes, then put them in a plastic bag, seal, and let them "sweat" for about 5 minutes.

Meanwhile, peel the onion and garlic cloves. Discard the thyme.

Take out the peppers and remove their stems, seeds, and skin (easiest done under running water). Put them in a blender with the garlic, onion, and lemon juice and whiz to a purée.

NOTE If you're going to make a soup, tip the red pepper purée into a pan and add about 2 cups vegetable stock to thin it down to the required consistency. Heat it through gently to serve.

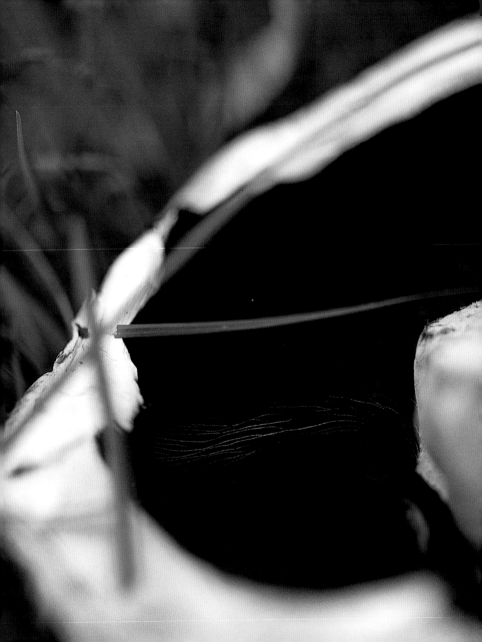

mushrooms

Scientists in North America and Europe are only just tapping into the wonders of mushrooms that have been used medicinally in Japan and China for millennia. They have isolated polysaccharides such as lentinan in shiitake, maitake, and reishi mushrooms, and shown them to power up the immune system dramatically. Not only are they strongly antibacterial and antiviral, but they have even been investigated for their potential in preventing and treating certain diseases, such as rheumatoid arthritis, cancer, and HIV. In addition to these powerful immune-boosting compounds, such mushrooms are also a good source of some B vitamins, iron, and zinc, which is needed for making energy and fighting off infections. Shiitake contain another active component, eritadenine, which has been shown to lower cholesterol. Even if you can't get these mushrooms fresh, dried ones store well and are a tasty addition to soups, casseroles, risottos, stir-fries, sauces, and even roasts. That way you still benefit from nature's synergy of all the compounds, some probably unknown.

hot & sour mushroom broth

THIS RECIPE IS BASED ON THE THAI SOUP *TOM YUM*. IT TAKES NO TIME TO MAKE, DESPITE THE LENGTHY INGREDIENTS LIST. IF FRESH SHIITAKE ARE UNOBTAINABLE, USE 2 OZ DRIED SHIITAKE INSTEAD—YOU'LL NEED TO MAKE SURE THE SOUP SIMMERS FOR LONG ENOUGH TO REHYDRATE THEM WELL. TO MAKE IT MORE FILLING, ADD A LARGE HANDFUL OF RICE NOODLES.

1/2 cup miso (**soy** paste)
6 cups boiling water
7 oz shiitake **mushrooms**
2 small, fresh, hot red
    chiles, seeded and sliced
1 lemongrass stalk, sliced
1-inch piece fresh **ginger**,
    peeled and grated
1-inch piece fresh galangal,
    peeled and sliced
    (optional)
3 dried kaffir lime leaves
4 **scallions**, trimmed
    and sliced
1 tbsp Thai fish sauce
1 tbsp tamari or soy sauce
1 tbsp **lime** juice
1 tbsp brown sugar or
    alternative equivalent
    (see page 10)
7 oz **spinach** leaves, washed
    and roughly torn
cilantro leaves, torn,
    for garnish

In a large pan, mix the miso paste with a little of the boiling water, then stir in the remaining water. Add the rest of the ingredients, except the spinach and cilantro, and bring to a boil. Immediately turn the heat down and simmer gently for about 10 minutes. Add the spinach at the last minute.

Serve the broth scattered with freshly torn cilantro. It tastes even better the next day.

mushroom baked chicken

THIS IS PRETTY MUCH THE ROAST CHICKEN STAPLE IN OUR HOUSE, USUALLY
COOKED IN AN OLD TERRACOTTA POT. YOU CAN COOK A WHOLE CHICKEN THE
SAME WAY.

1 **onion**, *peeled and sliced*
2 *heaped tbsp dried*
   seaweed
12 *shiitake* **mushrooms**,
   sliced
1/2-*inch piece fresh* **ginger**,
   peeled and grated
4 **chicken** *breast halves or*
   8 thighs
2 *tbsp tamari or soy sauce*
1/2 **lemon**
freshly ground black pepper

Preheat the oven to 375°F. Randomly scatter the
onion over the bottom of a large baking dish,
along with the crumbled dried seaweed, the
mushrooms, and the ginger. Put the chicken
pieces on top. Drizzle the tamari over and squeeze
the lemon over the chicken, then put the spent
lemon half in the dish. Season it all with pepper.

Pour in enough water to cover the mushrooms
and seaweed. Bake until the chicken pieces are
cooked through, 30–40 minutes.

Eat with Scented savory rice (page 67) and
steamed or stir-fried green veggies.

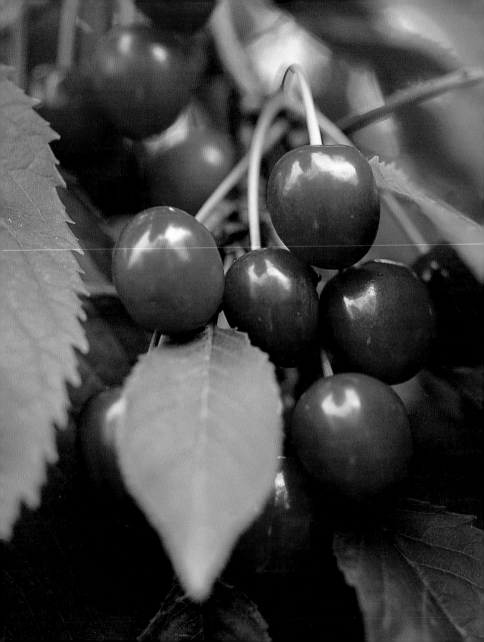

cherries

Cherries conjure up images of summer idyll, luxury, and the childhood memory of dangling double-stemmed fruit over my ears. It so happens that cherries are wonderfully good for you. As their deep, rich red color suggests, they are packed with powerful antioxidant compounds that support the body's immune system, fight arthritis, and can even help to protect against cancer and heart disease. Cherries are also rich in flavonoids called anthocyanins and in quercetin, which is strongly anti-inflammatory. Quercetin helps relieve painful inflammation of the joints, gout, and allergic reactions involving histamine; it's been shown to help reduce the formation of cataracts, too. The key antioxidants in cherries work alongside vitamin C to help ward off viruses (including the common cold) and to strengthen collagen, our cellular support structure that in effect holds our skin, blood vessels, and indeed our entire bodies together. Cherries are also a good source of several vitamins, including carotene, and minerals such as iron.

cherry chicken

YOU CAN EITHER REMOVE THE PITS FROM THE CHERRIES OR SAVE THE EFFORT AND
LEAVE THEM IN—JUST REMEMBER TO WARN EVERYONE BEFORE EATING!
IF FRESH CHERRIES ARE OUT OF SEASON, OPT FOR UNSWEETENED FROZEN ONES
INSTEAD. FOR AN ALCOHOL-FREE VERSION, USE WATER RATHER THAN WINE.

$1/2$ **onion**, peeled and sliced
1 tsp olive oil
8 star anise
4 **chicken** breasts with skin
    (or thighs or drumsticks)
2 tbsp tamari or soy sauce
1 tbsp **honey**
$1/2$ cup freshly squeezed
    orange juice
2 tbsp balsamic vinegar
$1/2$ cup red wine
$2^1/3$ cup **cherries**

Preheat the oven to 350°F. In a stovetop-to-oven casserole, soften the onion in the olive oil with the star anise. Add the chicken and cook until lightly colored, 2–3 minutes on each side. Stir in the tamari, honey, orange juice, balsamic vinegar, and wine. Bring to a boil, lower the heat, and simmer for 4–5 minutes.

Tip in the cherries and stir to mix. Cover and transfer to the oven to cook for 20 minutes, then squish the cherries into the sauce to make it darker and more flavorful. Bake, uncovered, until the chicken is tender, 20–25 minutes longer. Serve with brown rice and steamed green vegetables.

chocolatey cherries

THESE MAKE A TEMPTING LIGHT DESSERT, OR YOU CAN SERVE THEM WITH MINT TEA (OR COFFEE) AFTER DINNER. YOU NEED RIPE CHERRIES AND GOOD-QUALITY CHOCOLATE THAT'S AT LEAST 70% COCOA SOLIDS. USE HALF CHERRIES AND HALF STRAWBERRIES, IF PREFERRED.

1 lb **cherries**, with stems
7 oz dark **chocolate**

Rinse and dry the cherries. Line a baking sheet with parchment paper. Break up the chocolate into a heatproof bowl and rest the bowl on top of a pan of gently simmering water, making sure the base of the bowl doesn't touch the water. Leave until the chocolate is melted, then stir until smooth.

Holding it by the stem, dip each cherry into the melted chocolate to coat, then place on the lined baking sheet. Leave until the chocolate has set.

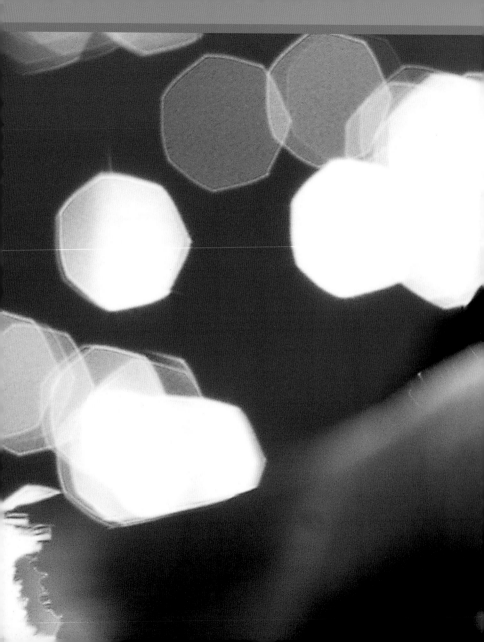

heart

The wonderfoods in this section are just a few of those that play a particularly important part in keeping all the various forms of cardiovascular disease (CVD) at bay. CVD is rife in the so-called "developed" countries, where we have acquired diets and lifestyles that leave us riddled with conditions that slowly kill us. Diseases of the heart and blood vessels, in the form of high blood pressure, thickening of the arteries, deposits in the arteries, inflammation in artery walls, blood clots, and high cholesterol, build up silently. These all clog up the arteries that supply the brain, heart, and other vital organs, resulting in heart attacks and strokes. All authorities on heart disease recognize that we do really have significant control over the degree to which any of these progress.

As you will see from the individual wonderfood entries, some help regulate blood pressure by contributing to the mineral balance in the body, acting as a diuretic, or relaxing blood vessels. Others help reduce the likelihood of blood clotting unnecessarily, which contributes to strokes and heart attacks. The buildup of cholesterol in the lining of blood vessels, particularly when it is oxidized and therefore damaged (see age introduction, page 170), is recognized as a major contributing factor to heart disease. As you will discover, many of these heart wonderfoods help to reduce the buildup of "harmful" cholesterol.

It is increasingly acknowledged that inflammation of the blood vessels underlies much CVD, and the wonderfoods here and others throughout the book help keep this down. Obviously, we need our blood to clot in certain situations, such as when we cut or graze ourselves. However, over-stickiness of the blood makes it more liable to form clots inside the body and these can be dangerous as they create blockages. This is particularly hazardous if this occurs in the brain (such as in a stroke) or in the blood supply to the heart.

The insidious nature of CVD is such that it creeps up on us and we only usually find out about it when it is established, so prevention is the key, as it is with most illnesses. That's not to say it's too late to make a difference if you have already been diagnosed with, say, high blood pressure or high cholesterol. Eating the wonderfoods here and throughout the book can play a key role, as it's indisputable that we can minimize our risk of succumbing to heart disease by eating healthily as well as exercising regularly, not smoking, not drinking excessive amounts of alcohol, and maintaining our ideal weight.

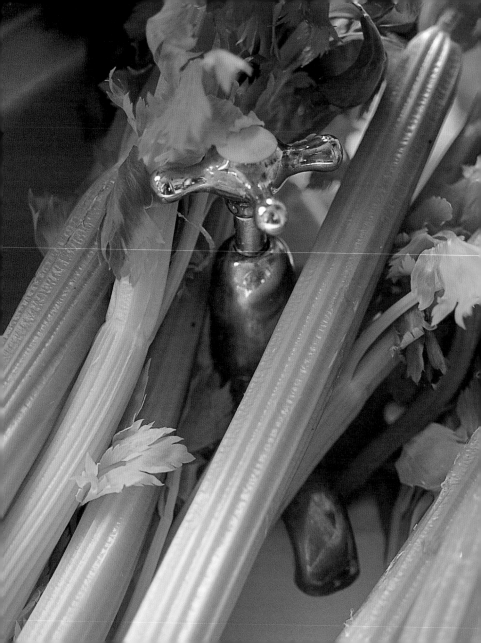

celery

Celery is as at home in an herbalist's apothecary as it is in the kitchen. Herbally, it is most widely used for helping to lower blood pressure on two fronts. One is because of its powerful diuretic action. The other is down to substances called phthalides, which help dilate blood vessels and that are, in general, relaxing. Celery is especially useful for people who suffer from water retention, because apart from its diuretic action, its potassium-sodium balance helps to regulate the body's fluids. Celery provides a decent amount of vitamin C, and valuable chemicals called coumarins, which have anti-cancer properties. Given that salt is linked to increasing blood pressure, it may seem somewhat contradictory that celery has a high organic sodium content that gives it a salty flavor and makes it useful for dislodging calcified buildups in the joints. Strongly alkaline, celery is detoxifying and calming on the digestive system, and for many years it has been traditionally used to treat rheumatic and arthritic conditions, as well as gout.

crisp bean salad

THIS IS A STAPLE LUNCH IN OUR HOUSE—IT'S EASY TO MAKE AND VERY PORTABLE,
TOO. YOU COULD VARY THE FLAVOR BY USING DIFFERENT OILS OR HERBS, SUCH AS
TOASTED SESAME OIL AND CILANTRO WITH A DASH OF HOT PEPPER SAUCE.

2 cans (14 oz each) **beans**
(pinto, cannellini
or mixed), drained
and rinsed
2 medium **tomatoes**,
roughly chopped
4 **scallions**, trimmed
and sliced
4 **celery** stalks, finely sliced
pinch of sea salt
2 tbsp olive oil
1 tbsp **lemon** juice
2 heaped tbsp finely
chopped **parsley**

In a large bowl, mix the beans with all the other
ingredients. That's it!

chicken & arugula salad

THIS MAKES A GOOD WEEKEND SUMMER LUNCH. YOU CAN COOK THE CHICKEN
BREASTS IN ADVANCE TO PILE ON TOP OF THE SALAD ANY TIME.

4 skinless, boneless **chicken**
  breast halves
1 tbsp pesto
4 handfuls of arugula leaves
4 **celery** stalks, finely sliced
8 cherry **tomatoes**, halved
1 **avocado**, peeled, pitted,
  and cubed
FOR THE VINAIGRETTE
2 tbsp balsamic vinegar
1 heaped tsp Dijon mustard
6 tbsp olive oil
freshly ground black pepper

Preheat the oven to 400°F. Spread the pesto all
over the chicken breasts and lay them in a baking
dish. Add enough water to just cover the bottom
of the dish. Bake until the chicken is cooked
through, about 25 minutes; test with a skewer—
the juices should run clear.

Meanwhile, assemble the salad ingredients. To
make the vinaigrette, put the balsamic vinegar and
mustard in a lidded jar and shake well, then add
the olive oil and pepper and shake again.

When the chicken is cooked, pile the salad
ingredients onto four plates and drizzle about
1 tbsp vinaigrette over each portion. Slice the
chicken breasts and arrange on top of the salad.
Serve at once.

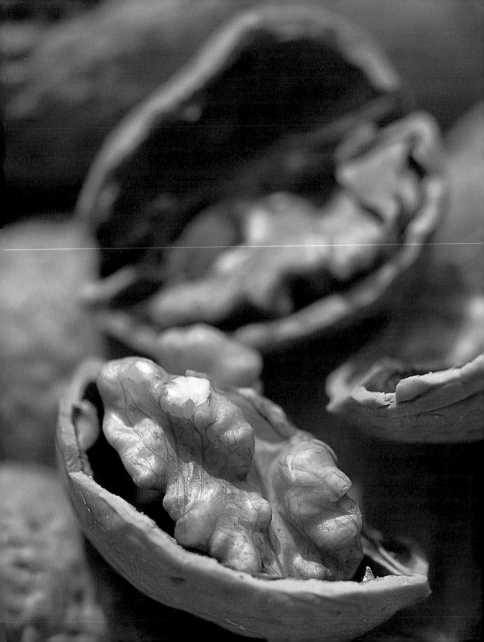

walnuts

Apparently walnuts were eaten by Jupiter and other gods, who would have gained from more than just their taste. These nuts are loaded with essential fatty acids (EFAs), particularly the omega-6s, but also omega-3s and monounsaturates (like olive oil). Omega-3s have a host of benefits for the cardiovascular system. They lower LDL cholesterol (the "bad" type), improving its ratio to HDL (the "good" type), lower lipoprotein A (another "baddie"), make blood less likely to clot, and increase the elasticity of arteries. Arginine, an amino acid in walnuts, also helps blood vessels relax, reducing the chance of high blood pressure. Antioxidant chemicals such as ellagic acid protect cholesterol from oxidative damage, as well as conferring anti-cancer properties. EFAs also make for better nerve transmission (needed for good memory and moods), keep skin smooth, and calm inflammation in conditions such as asthma, arthritis, eczema, and psoriasis. On top of all this, walnuts contain the minerals copper, manganese, iron, and zinc, as well as fiber and B vitamins.

pear & walnut sweet polenta

THIS IS AN UNUSUAL, VERY EASY "TART" THAT CAN BE EATEN AS A DESSERT OR EVEN AT TEATIME.

1/2 cup **apple** juice
1³/₄ cups water
2 tbsp **honey** or maple syrup
3 ripe but firm **pears**, cored and sliced
1¹/₄ cups cornmeal
1 tsp butter
a little olive oil for brushing
about 20 **walnut** halves, broken up
FOR SERVING
²/₃ cup plain **yogurt**
1/2 tsp vanilla extract, or to taste

Preheat the oven to 350°F. Pour the apple juice and water into a large saucepan, add the honey, and bring to a boil. Turn down the heat and add the pear slices. Simmer for 6–7 minutes, then remove the pears with a slotted spoon and set aside.

Slowly add the cornmeal to the liquid in the pan, whisking constantly to avoid it getting lumpy. Add the butter as you whisk. Continue to cook, stirring regularly, until the polenta is very thick and comes away from the sides of the pan easily, about 10 minutes.

Rub the bottom of a 9-inch tart pan with olive oil, pour in the polenta, and bake for 30 minutes. Lay the pear slices on the polenta, scatter the walnuts over the top, and bake for 15 minutes longer. Meanwhile, flavor the yogurt with a few drops of vanilla extract to taste.

Cut the "tart" into slices and eat warm, with the vanilla-flavoured yogurt or sour cream.

savory walnut pâté

THIS CAN BE EATEN ON CRACKERS OR TOAST, OR EVEN WITH CRUDITÉS AS A DIP.

*1 heaped cup **walnuts** pieces*
*handful of **parsley**, plus*
sprigs for garnish
5 oz feta cheese, crumbled
½ cup water
*1 small **garlic** clove, peeled*
1 tsp ground coriander
few shakes of cayenne
pepper
a little olive oil

Put the walnuts and parsley in a blender and pulse until the nuts are ground. Then add the feta, water, garlic, coriander, and cayenne, and whiz briefly until smooth.

Spoon into a serving dish, drizzle with a little olive oil, and top with a few parsley sprigs.

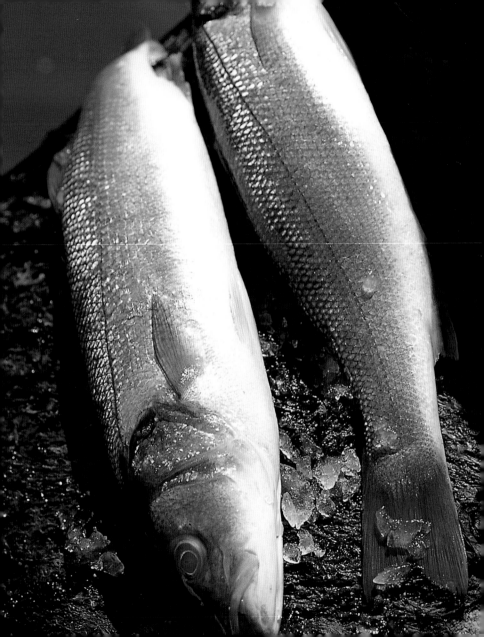

fish

Fish are not only heart food, but a total wonderfood. All are an excellent source of protein, and oily fish—fresh tuna, salmon, sardines, herring, mackerel, trout—are rich sources of the omega-3 essential fatty acids (EFAs), DHA (docosahexaenoic acid), and EPA (eicosapentenoic acid). These fats are renowned for reducing heart attacks and factors that contribute to cardiovascular disease, such as blood clotting and high blood pressure. EFAs are integrated into cell membranes, so not only do they make your skin smooth, they also help the function of every single cell. DHA is especially important in the brain and nervous system, helping to improve learning, to combat age-related memory decline, and to enhance mood. EFAs also have powerful anti-inflammatory properties, making them useful in conditions such as arthritis, asthma, and eczema. Fish is a source of sulfur, a valuable mineral for detoxification. It also contains choline, a B-vitamin family member, needed for healthy cell membranes and for the formation of the body's own memory messenger, the neurotransmitter acetylcholine.

fish kebabs

YOU CAN VARY THESE KEBABS BY CHOOSING DIFFERENT FISH, OR PERHAPS
CHICKEN OR LAMB, AND OTHER VEGETABLES SUCH AS PAR-BOILED CHUNKS OF
CORN-ON-THE-COB OR ROASTED SWEET POTATOES.

*7 oz **monkfish** fillet, cubed*
*7 oz **salmon** fillet, cubed*
*4 sea scallops, shucked and
    cleaned*
*4 large, raw shrimp, peeled,
    but with last tail section
    left on and deveined*
*1 red **bell pepper**, seeded
    and cut into squares*
*1 yellow **bell pepper**,
    deseeded and cut
    into squares*
*2 zucchini, sliced into
    ¹/₂-inch chunks*
FOR THE MARINADE
*juice of 3 **limes***
freshly ground black pepper
3 tbsp olive oil
*³/₄ tsp ground **turmeric***
³/₄ tsp ground cumin
1 tsp hot pepper sauce

In a large dish, mix all the marinade ingredients
together. Add the cubed fish, scallops, and shrimp,
turning to coat them well. Let marinate for about
20 minutes.

Preheat the broiler. Remove the fish and
shellfish from the dish, reserving the marinade.
Thread them onto four skewers, alternating with
the vegetables. Broil the kebabs until the fish is
cooked, about 3 minutes on each side, basting
them with the marinade as you turn them.

Serve on brown rice (cooked in fish stock
rather than water for extra flavor) with a
Wonderfoods green salad (page 111).

NOTE If you use wooden rather than metal
skewers, you will need to soak them in advance
to prevent them from scorching under the broiler.

nellie fish

THIS WAY OF COOKING FISH IS A STAPLE AT THE HOME OF MY FRIENDS, NELLIE AND MICHAEL. IT'S MY FAVORITE WAY OF COOKING HALIBUT, ALTHOUGH I OFTEN USE HADDOCK FOR A CHEAPER OPTION.

16–20 cherry **tomatoes**
2 tbsp olive oil
8 **garlic** cloves (unpeeled)
2 fresh, hot red or green
    chiles
1 tbsp tamari or soy sauce
4 fillets of any **fish** you like,
    each about 6 oz

Preheat the oven to 400°F. Put the cherry tomatoes, olive oil, garlic cloves, whole chiles, and tamari in a large baking dish, toss well, and bake until the tomatoes are slightly wrinkled, about 20 minutes.

Add the fish fillets, swishing them around in the dish and turning to coat them on both sides with the mixture. Bake until the fish is cooked, 15–20 minutes, depending on the size of the fillets. Discard the chiles.

Eat with a Wonderfoods green salad (page 111) and boiled buckwheat, squeezing out the garlic onto the fish and tomatoes as you eat them.

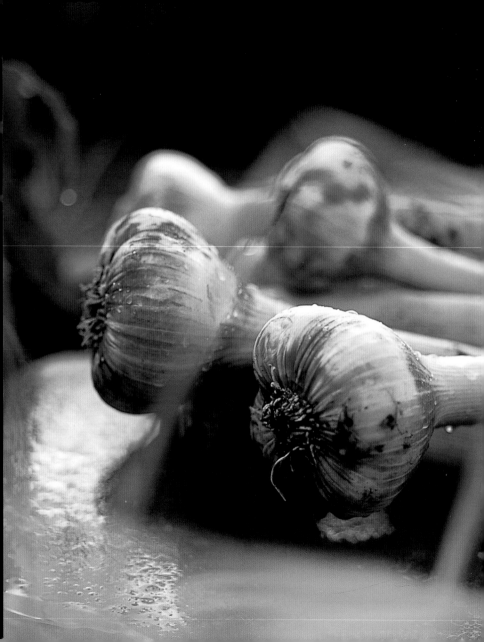

garlic

In Asia, ancient records show that garlic has been valued for thousands of years as a potent medicine, with powers as far reaching as an aphrodisiac, a purifier, healer, and strength-builder. Heartwise, garlic is a megastar. It helps prevent hardening of arteries, reduces LDL cholesterol and blood fats while increasing HDL, deters the clumping of blood cells, lowers blood pressure, and helps prevent harmful oxidative damage to cholesterol. Many of its benefits derive from sulfur compounds, such as allicin, that are also powerful detoxifiers for the liver and lymph system as well as anti-inflammatories. Garlic is also a powerful antibiotic, helping clear bacterial, fungal, worm, and amoebic infections in the digestive tract. This property, plus its immune-boosting role and decongestant effect, enables garlic to ward off viral and other infections throughout the body, including coughs and colds. It also helps to protect against cancer. To get the most, healthwise, from garlic, it's best eaten raw—in salads or mixed into dishes after they have been cooked.

som tam

THIS IS A MILD VERSION OF ONE OF MY FAVORITE DISHES. TRADITIONALLY FROM NORTHEAST THAILAND, IT'S MADE TO ORDER WITH A MORTAR AND PESTLE AT STREET STALLS AND SERVED WITH STICKY RICE AND GRILLED CHICKEN. VISIT YOUR LOCAL ASIAN MARKET TO GET THE INGREDIENTS. IF YOU CAN'T FIND GREEN PAPAYA, USE HALF A HEAD OF WHITE CABBAGE INSTEAD.

2 **garlic** cloves
1 fresh Thai chile
1 tbsp coconut palm sugar
    (jaggery)
2 heaped tbsp roasted
    peanuts (not salted)
10 green beans, sliced
4 cherry **tomatoes**
1/2 green **papaya**, peeled,
    seeded, and finely
    shredded
juice of 2 **limes**
1 tbsp tamarind concentrate,
    diluted with 2 tsp water
1 tbsp Thai fish sauce

Using a mortar and pestle, crush the garlic, chile, palm sugar, and peanuts together. Add the beans and tomatoes, pounding all the time. Bit by bit, add the shredded papaya, still pounding.

Slowly add the lime juice, then the tamarind juice and fish sauce, continuing to pound. Taste and add a little more lime and tamarind if you want a sharper flavor. Eat immediately, with grilled chicken and rice.

roasted garlic & tomato soup

THIS IS A VERY DENSE, WARMING SOUP, ALTHOUGH YOU COULD THIN IT DOWN
WITH EXTRA STOCK OR WATER IF YOU WANT SOMETHING LIGHTER.

2 **garlic** bulbs, broken into
   cloves (unpeeled)
10 medium-large **tomatoes**
splash of olive oil
2 cups vegetable or chicken
   stock
10–12 **basil** leaves
2 tbsp **lemon** juice
1/2 tsp cayenne pepper

Preheat the oven to 400°F. Toss the garlic cloves
and tomatoes in a splash of olive oil in a baking
dish. Roast them for 40 minutes.

Peel away the skins from the roasted garlic
cloves and tomatoes, then put them in a large
saucepan with the stock, basil leaves, lemon juice,
and cayenne. Bring to a boil, then whiz it all up
using an immersion blender.

Serve the soup hot, with chunks of rye bread.

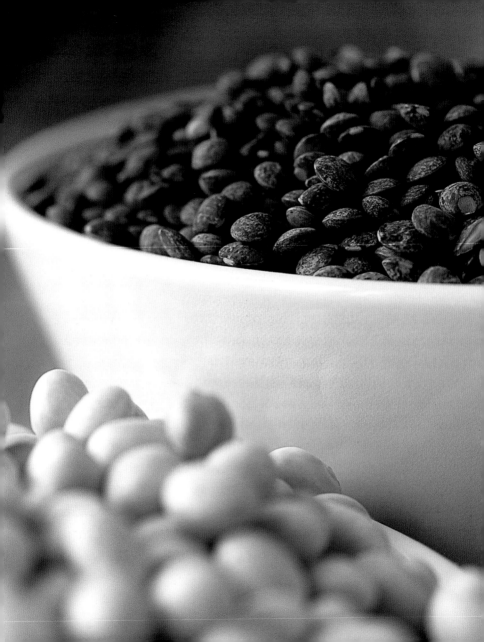

lentils & beans

Not the easiest of foods to digest, beans and lentils have a valid reputation for inducing wind, but they have hidden talents. Scientists have shown that eating such high-fiber foods dramatically lowers the risk of heart disease. One reason is that fiber binds with cholesterol in the gut and ferries it out of the body. Plenty of fiber also means that blood-sugar levels don't rise rapidly after eating, keeping insulin from shooting up—especially useful for people with diabetes or other blood-sugar problems. Rising insulin levels stimulate the production of cholesterol, and people with diabetes have a greater risk of cardiovascular disease. Beans contain folic acid, which helps lower the chemical homocysteine, high levels of which are linked to heart disease, Alzheimer's, and depression. All in all, beans and lentils are a low-fat, low-calorie, dense source of fiber, protein, vitamins, and minerals. To reduce their wind potential, soak lentils and beans well before cooking and then use fresh water to boil, or cook them with some kombu seaweed and ginger, or sprout them (see page 110).

warm puy lentil salad

YOU CAN EAT THIS SALAD WARM OR COLD. THE COLD-PRESSED SUNFLOWER OIL
ADDS A NUTTY TOUCH. IF YOU CAN'T GET HOLD OF IT, DOUBLE THE AMOUNT OF
OLIVE OIL RATHER THAN USING REGULAR SUPERMARKET SUNFLOWER OIL.

*2 cups Puy **lentils***
*3 medium **tomatoes***
*3 **scallions**, trimmed and*
*   finely sliced*
*10–12 **basil** leaves,*
*   roughly torn*
1 tbsp olive oil
1 tbsp cold-pressed
*   **sunflower oil***
2 tsp balsamic vinegar
freshly ground black pepper
pinch of salt

Wash the lentils and put them in a large saucepan. Add water to cover generously and bring to a boil. Lower the heat and let simmer until the lentils are tender, about 30 minutes.

While they are cooking, drop the tomatoes into the pan for a minute to loosen the skins, then remove with a slotted spoon and peel away the skins. Roughly chop the tomato flesh.

Drain the lentils well and toss them with the tomatoes and all the other ingredients. Serve with a Wonderfoods green salad (page 111).

fruity baked beans

THIS IS INSPIRED BY A RECIPE IN THE VEGETARIAN MOOSEWOOD COOKBOOK BY
MOLLIE KATZEN. I SOMETIMES ADD LEAN, CHUNKY BACON TO MAKE IT EVEN
HEARTIER FOR SUPPER ON A WINTER'S NIGHT.

*3 **onions**, peeled and sliced*
1 tbsp olive oil
2 tsp ground coriander
1 tsp smoked paprika
1 tsp cayenne pepper
*2 large, tart cooking **apples**,*
*   peeled, cored, and cut*
*   into ¹/₂-inch chunks*
*4 medium **tomatoes**,*
*   peeled and chopped*
*8 **garlic** cloves, peeled*
*   and crushed*
6 tbsp cider vinegar
*¹/₄ cup molasses or **honey***
2 star anise
3 cans (14 oz each)
*   cannellini **beans**,*
*   drained*

Preheat the oven to 350°F. In a large saucepan,
soften the onions in the olive oil with the ground
coriander, paprika, and cayenne pepper for about
10 minutes. Add the apples, tomatoes, garlic,
vinegar, molasses, and star anise. Stir and cook
for 4–5 minutes before adding the beans.

Transfer to a casserole or bean pot, cover, and
cook in the oven for 1 hour.

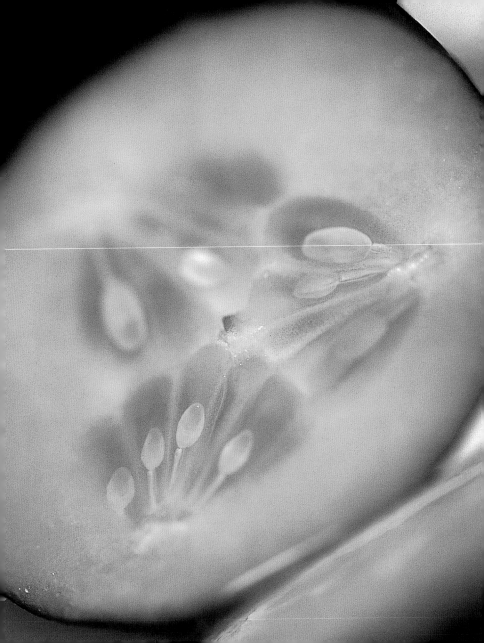

cucumber

This water-laden member of the gourd family (related to summer and winter squashes and watermelon) has been popular since ancient times, not just as a food, but also for its skin-healing properties. Its high water and balanced mineral content makes cucumber one of the best-known diuretics—it helps the body eliminate water, which in turn keeps blood pressure down. This "flushing" of water through the kidneys also means that cucumber is a good detoxifier, helping the body eliminate waste products. A high water intake also helps keep the bowels moving well. The advice to drink however many glasses of water a day often doesn't take into account the water in foods: if you eat plenty of fruits and vegetables like cucumbers, you don't need to drink quite so much water. Cucumbers are rich in silica, a mineral needed for healthy skin, bone, and all connective tissues in the body, and also the somewhat obscure mineral molybdenum, which is needed for detoxification. Cucumbers also provide a range of other nutrients, such as vitamin C, potassium, magnesium, and fiber.

cucumber fettuccine salad

THIS SALAD GOES WELL WITH CARROT FELAFEL (PAGE 183) AND IS A GOOD
ACCOMPANIMENT TO JERUSALEM CHICKEN (PAGE 34). IT DOESN'T CONTAIN PASTA,
BUT TAKES ITS NAME FROM THE FINE-CUT CUCUMBER RIBBONS.

1 long English **cucumber**
1 heaped tbsp chopped
mint
2 heaped tbsp chopped
parsley
2 tbsp **lemon** *juice*
2 tbsp olive oil
1 cup cottage cheese
freshly ground black pepper
pinch of sea salt

Using a swivel potato peeler, pare the cucumber
into long, fine ribbons, dropping them onto a
clean kitchen towel. Pat them to remove some of
the liquid. Discard the outer skin pieces, then tip
into a large bowl. Add all the other ingredients and
toss lightly to mix, then serve.

spicy tuna & cucumber salad

A FAIL-SAFE RECIPE. USE ANY FISH YOU FANCY.

4 fresh **tuna** steaks, each
   about 5 oz
FOR THE MARINADE
1 tbsp hot pepper sauce
1 tbsp **lemon** juice
1 tbsp olive oil
2 **garlic** cloves, peeled
   and crushed
FOR THE SALAD
1 long English **cucumber**,
   cut into ¼-inch-thick
   slices
1 red **bell pepper**, cored,
   seeded, and finely sliced
2 tbsp **lemon** juice
2 tbsp olive oil
1 heaped tbsp chopped
   cilantro
2 tsp tamari or soy sauce

Combine the marinade ingredients in a shallow
dish, add the tuna steaks, and turn to coat. Let the
fish marinate for about 30 minutes.

Meanwhile, make the salad. Toss all the
ingredients together in a bowl, then divide among
four plates.

Preheat a ridged, castiron grill pan. Sear the
tuna steaks until cooked to your taste, about
2 minutes on each side. Lay the tuna steaks on
top of the salad and serve immediately.

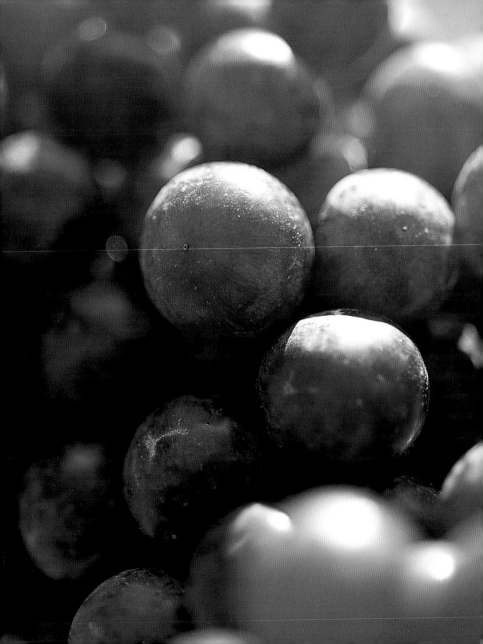

grapes

In ancient literature you'll find tales of grapes, their symbolism, and their association with wine and hedonism. Today, scientific literature abounds on their remarkable health benefits. Grapes contain antioxidant flavonoid compounds that not only protect against heart disease, but also cancer and aging. Saponins, pterostilbene, resveratrol, and other substances contribute in many ways to cutting the risk of heart disease by reducing platelet clumping and blood clots, dropping blood pressure, lowering LDL cholesterol, inhibiting the oxidation of LDL, relaxing blood vessels, preventing the heart muscle from stiffening, and reducing inflammation, which is increasingly recognized as a cause of cardiovascular problems. Resveratrol in particular is exciting scientists as a cancer-preventative agent. The water and fiber in grapes makes them useful against constipation and for detoxifying the gut and liver. Get the benefits from grapes themselves and grape juice (especially red), rather than wine, as the alcohol and preservatives can trigger migraines and other problems.

scallop, grape & grapefruit salad

THIS IS A FINE, REFRESHING SALAD. IF SCALLOPS AREN'T AVAILABLE, YOU CAN
SUBSTITUTE SHRIMP OR BITE-SIZED PIECES OF CHICKEN.

16–20 red **grapes**, washed
1 pink **grapefruit**
4 handfuls of **watercress**,
    washed
16 sea scallops, shucked
    and cleaned
a little olive oil
FOR THE DRESSING
¼ cup **grapefruit** juice
1 tbsp olive oil
1 tbsp sweet chile sauce

Halve the grapes and remove the seeds. Peel and segment the grapefruit, discarding all membrane and pith. Arrange the grapes, grapefruit, and watercress on four plates.

Shake the dressing ingredients together in a lidded jar.

Preheat a ridged, castiron grill pan and oil it very lightly. Sear the scallops in the hot pan for about 1 minute each side, then lay them on top of the salad. Drizzle a little dressing over each portion and eat immediately.

frosted grapes

handful of green **grapes**, *washed*
handful of red **grapes**, *washed*
few splashes of sweet wine, brandy, or apple juice

Lay the grapes on a tray or in a large plastic container and put them in the freezer overnight. Get them out of the freezer and eat them right away, drizzled with a little sweet wine, brandy, or apple juice.

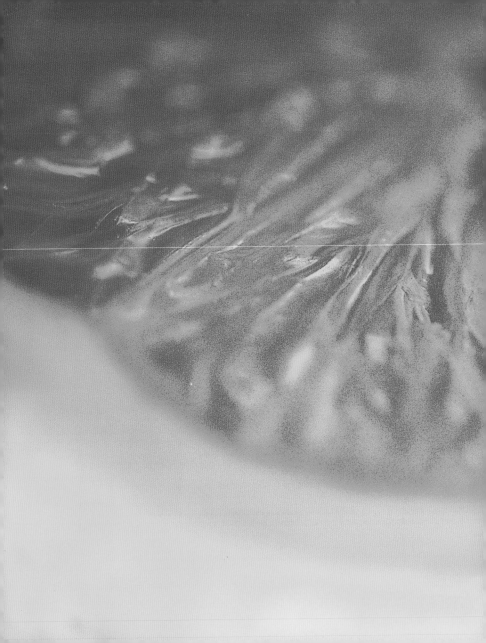

reference

wonderfoods week

YOU COULD EASILY GO THROUGH AN ENTIRE WEEK EATING MEALS MADE UP OF
WONDERFOODS. HERE'S JUST A SAMPLE IDEA OF HOW TO DO IT.

	Breakfast	*Lighter Meal*	*Main Meal*	*Dessert*
Mon	Honeyed granola (page 38)	Papaya & shrimp salad (page 54)	Lemongrass turkey skewers (page 210)	Apple custard tart (page 51)
Tues	Black-currant smoothie (page 238)	Artichoke heart pizzas (page 107)	Soba noodles & salmon (page 75)	Mango with coconut rice (page 31)
Wed	Scrambled eggs with watercress (page 203)	Marinated red onion & beet salad (page 90)	Jerusalem chicken (page 34)	Black currant & apricot slice (page 239)
Thurs	Spiced apricots (page 174)	Frittata tricolore (page 150)	Mackerel with apple purée (page 50)	Blueberry cheesecake (page 178)
Fri	Mango incognito (page 179)	Kiwi & figs with prosciutto (page 190)	White bean mash (page 199)	Roasted pears with lime & ginger (page 79)
Sat	Fruity oatmeal (page 223)	Broccoli-polenta quiche (page 227)	Seed-crusted monkfish in prosciutto (page 147)	Orange almond torte (page 118)
Sun	Buckwheat crêpes (page 74)	Hot & sour mushroom broth (page 258)	Moroccan lamb (page 194)	Pan-grilled papaya with lime honey (page 55)

wonderfoods contacts

FIND LOCAL FARM SHOPS AND ORGANIC DELIVERY SERVICES BY RECOMMENDATION OR BY SEARCHING THE WEB OR YOUR BOOKSHOP FOR AN ORGANIC DIRECTORY. OTHERWISE, JUST CHOOSE THE FRESHEST, BEST QUALITY PRODUCE THAT YOU CAN FIND AND AFFORD, IDEALLY LOCALLY PRODUCED AND ORGANIC.

Natalie Savona's nutrition work

For information, visit www.nataliesavona.com

Slow food

International organization aiming to preserve artisanal foods and regional traditions. www.slowfood.com

Farmers' markets

A website of the USDA organization that promotes farmers' markets throughout the US. Markets listed state by state, with locations, times, and contacts. www.ams.usda.gov/farmersmarkets/

OTHER READING

The Whole Foods Companion Dianne Onstad (Chelsea Green Publishing, Vermont)
Herbal Deni Brown (Pavilion Books, London)
Cabbages & Kings Jonathan Roberts (HarperCollins, London)
The Kitchen Shrink Natalie Savona (Duncan Baird Publishing, London)
The Big Book of Juices and Smoothies Natalie Savona (Duncan Baird Publishing, London)
Books by Alice Waters, Hugh Fearnley-Whittingstall.

wonderfoods nutrient sources

NUTRIENTS PLAY A VITAL PART IN ALL THE WORKINGS OF THE HUMAN BODY,
MAINTAINING GOOD HEALTH AND FIGHTING DISEASE. HERE IS A SUMMARY OF THE
ROLES OF KEY NUTRIENTS AND WONDERFOODS YOU CAN EAT TO OBTAIN THEM.

Vitamin	Nutrient for...
Vitamin A/beta-carotene	Antioxidant; protects skin and "internal skin"—lungs, gut; eyes; reproduction; immunity
Vitamin B1 (thiamin)	Energy production; nervous system; carbohydrate processing
Vitamin B2 (riboflavin)	Energy; skin; nervous system
Vitamin B3 (niacin)	Energy; nervous system; moods; blood-sugar balance; cholesterol balance; stress response; hormonal balance
Vitamin B5 (pantothenic acid)	Energy production; body's stress response; regeneration of cells; anti-inflammatory; immunity
Vitamin B6	Energy production; nervous system; moods and brain power; hormone balance; protein digestion; immunity
Vitamin B12	Brain and nervous system; red blood cell formation; lowers toxic homocysteine; cellular energy and reproduction
Folic acid (folate)	Brain and nervous system, especially in fetal growth; cellular energy and reproduction; moods; cardiovascular health; red blood cell formation; lowers toxic homocysteine
Biotin	Energy production; fat and amino acid processing; skin, nails, and hair
Vitamin C (ascorbic acid)	Antioxidant; collagen formation: skin, blood vessels, and gums; aids iron absorption; immunity; helps protect against illness, allergies, pollution, stress, and aging; anti-inflammatory

Wonderfood sources

Apricot, broccoli, carrot, kale, spinach, sweet potato, pumpkin, melon, watermelon, egg

Beans, sunflower seeds, fish, brown rice, oats, rye, quinoa, buckwheat, molasses, chicken, turkey, lamb, egg

Almonds, walnuts, Brazil nuts, oats, spinach, yogurt, egg, fish, chicken, turkey, lamb

Chicken, turkey, lamb, fish, seeds, beans, lentils, soy, yogurt

Egg, fish, chicken, turkey, lamb, brown rice, oats, rye, quinoa, buckwheat, lentils, soy

Chicken, turkey, lamb, fish, almonds, walnuts, Brazil nuts, brown rice, oats, rye, quinoa, buckwheat, avocado, banana, seeds, beans, lentils

Eggs, fish, chicken, turkey, lamb, yogurt

All fruits, beans, lentils, soy, spinach, kale, parsley, oats, rye, quinoa, buckwheat

Egg, brown rice, oats, rye, quinoa, buckwheat, lentils, fish, seeds

Black currants, berries, broccoli, cabbage, citrus fruit, sweet pepper, kale, kiwi fruit, papaya, spinach, tomato, watercress

Vitamin	Nutrient for...
Vitamin D	Helps calcium usage; bones and teeth; some cancer protection
Vitamin E	Antioxidant; immunity; helps protect skin, brain, circulation, and hormones; cardiovascular system
Vitamin K	Blood clotting; bone building

Mineral	Nutrient for...
Calcium	Bone building; muscle contraction and relaxation; regular heart beat; blood clotting; nerve transmission
Chromium	Processing of carbohydrates and sugars; blood-sugar balance; works with insulin
Copper	Production and transport of red blood cells; iron absorption; antioxidant
Iodine	Forms part of thyroid hormone
Iron	Forms part of hemoglobin, i.e. helps transport oxygen; other uses include cell reproduction
Magnesium	Energy production; hormone balance; muscle and nerve function; cardiovascular health; blood-sugar balance; works with calcium
Manganese	Antioxidant; energy production; nerves and brain; blood sugar balance; thyroid function
Potassium	Works with sodium to control fluid balance, blood pressure, nerves, muscles
Selenium	Antioxidant; works with vitamin E; immunity; cardiovascular health; anti-inflammatory

Wonderfood sources

Fish, egg, yogurt

Almonds, walnuts, Brazil nuts, seeds and seed oils, egg

Alfalfa sprouts, kale, parsley, spinach, broccoli, cauliflower, green tea

Wonderfood sources

Almonds, Brazil nuts, walnuts, seeds, kale, spinach, broccoli, canned fish, yogurt, molasses

Chicken, turkey, lamb, egg, fish, brown rice, oats, rye, quinoa, buckwheat, walnuts, almonds, Brazil nuts

Fish, walnuts, almonds, Brazil nuts, seeds, oats, rye, quinoa, buckwheat

Fish, seaweed

Egg, lamb, chicken, turkey, fish, prunes, seeds, seaweed, spinach, kale, brown rice, oats, rye, quinoa, buckwheat

Brown rice, oats, rye, quinoa, buckwheat, seeds, almonds, Brazil nuts, walnuts, molasses

Avocado, berries, buckwheat, ginger, hazelnuts, oats, seaweed, spinach

Avocado, banana, citrus fruit, lentils, nuts, sardines, spinach, whole grains

Fish, seeds, brown rice, oats, rye, quinoa, buckwheat, walnuts, Brazil nuts, almonds

Mineral	Nutrient for...
Sulfur	Antioxidant; helps liver detoxification; collagen production; skin, hair, nails
Zinc	Antioxidant; growth and development; all protein production; energy production; hormone production and balance; digestion; sexual function; skin health

Other essential nutrients	Nutrient for...
Essential fatty acids	As their name suggests, these are types of fats that the body cannot produce itself, so they must be obtained from food. They are needed for good hormone balance; healthy nerve and brain activities; smooth skin; cardiovascular health; they also have anti-inflammatory properties.
Protein	These are molecules made up of amino acids linked together in a particular order specified by a gene. They are needed for the structure, function, and regulation of all the body's cells and organs. Hormones, neurotransmitters, enzymes, transporters, and immune cells are proteins.
Carbohydrate	These are mainly sugars and starches that the body breaks down into glucose, a simple sugar used as fuel for the cells to make energy. They are found in sugar, all cereals, the wonderfoods listed opposite, and other foods. The body also uses carbohydrate to make a substance called glycogen, which is stored in the body for future use.

Wonderfood sources

Cabbage, egg, fish, garlic, onion

Egg, fish, chicken, turkey, lamb, seeds, yogurt

Wonderfood sources

Fish, seeds, nuts

Egg, fish, turkey, chicken, lamb, yogurt, soy, nuts, seeds, beans, lentils

All fruit and vegetables, rice, buckwheat, oats, quinoa, rye, sweet potato, lentils, beans, honey

wonderfoods therapy

WE'RE ALL AWARE OF THE EFFECT THAT SOME FOODS AND DRINKS HAVE ON US: DRINK COFFEE AND YOU FEEL MORE ALERT, EAT TOO MUCH CAKE AND YOU FEEL BLOATED! AND THE SAME GOES FOR MANY COMMON AILMENTS—CERTAIN FOODS MAKE THEM WORSE, WHILE SOME WONDERFOODS CAN HELP FIGHT, RELIEVE, OR PREVENT THE SYMPTOMS. EATING THE FOODS SUGGESTED IS NOT INTENDED AS A REPLACEMENT FOR MEDICAL ADVICE.

	Wonderfoods to eat
Acne	All fruit and vegetable fiber, oats, rye, brown rice, beans, lentils, beets, greens such as spinach, broccoli, watercress, and kale, parsley, almonds, avocado, strawberries, mango, pumpkin, sweet potato, carrot, garlic, seeds, yogurt
Anemia	Greens such as spinach, broccoli, watercress, and kale, parsley, beets, strawberries, kiwi fruit, citrus fruit, fish, egg, turkey, chicken, lamb, molasses
Arthritis	All fresh fruit and vegetables, especially strawberries, blueberries, cherries, carrot, broccoli, watercress, kiwi fruit, apricot, and pineapple, garlic, ginger, seeds and seed oils, fish, walnuts, Brazil nuts, prunes, turmeric, cinnamon
Asthma	All fresh fruit and vegetables, especially blueberries, cherries, carrot, sweet pepper, broccoli, watercress, and apricot, ginger, garlic, seeds and seed oils, fish, onion, pumpkin, sweet potato, walnuts
Bladder infection	Blueberries, watermelon, melon, broccoli, cherries, strawberries, kiwi fruit, citrus fruit, garlic, yogurt
Boils	Blueberries, strawberries, watermelon, melon, kiwi fruit, citrus fruit, garlic, spinach, broccoli, watercress, kale, parsley, beets, artichoke, avocado, cucumber, almonds, mango, pumpkin, sweet potato, carrot

Bronchitis	Apricot, sweet pepper, watercress, watermelon, melon, blueberries, broccoli, strawberries, cherries, kiwi fruit, citrus fruit, garlic, seeds, pumpkin, sweet potato, onion, cloves
Burns, cuts & bruises	Apricot, sweet pepper, carrot, watercress, watermelon, melon, broccoli, strawberries, cherries, kiwi fruit, citrus fruit, garlic, seeds, mango, avocado, almonds, pumpkin, sweet potato
Candidiasis	Oats, rye, brown rice, beans, lentils, spinach, broccoli, watercress, kale, parsley, artichoke, beets, asparagus, dandelion, cucumber, yogurt, garlic
Cardiovascular disease	All fruit and vegetable fiber, oats, rye, brown rice, beans, lentils, broccoli, strawberries, cherries, kiwi fruit, citrus fruit, celery, garlic, cucumber, grapes, seeds and seed oils, fish, turmeric, walnuts, Brazil nuts, prunes
Chronic fatigue	Greens such as spinach, broccoli, watercress, and kale, parsley, strawberries, kiwi fruit, citrus fruit, yogurt, egg, lamb, turkey, chicken, seeds and seed oils, fish, oats, buckwheat, seaweed
Cold sores	Watermelon, melon, broccoli, blueberries, strawberries, cherries, kiwi fruit, citrus fruit, garlic, carrot, sweet pepper, watercress, apricot, avocado, mango, pumpkin, sweet potato, garlic
Colitis	Watermelon, melon, broccoli, blueberries, strawberries, kiwi fruit, citrus fruit, garlic, carrot, sweet pepper, watercress, kale, apricot, pineapple, papaya, seeds and seed oils, fish, turmeric, cardamom
Common cold and flu	All fresh fruit and vegetables, especially blueberries, carrot, apricot, broccoli, watercress, strawberries, kiwi fruit, pumpkin, sweet potato, onion, and pineapple, ginger, garlic, seeds and seed oils, fish, Brazil nuts, cloves, cinnamon

Constipation	All fresh fruit and vegetables, prunes, oats, rye, brown rice, beans, lentils, seeds and seed oils, plenty of water and vegetable juices, dandelion, beets, artichoke, cucumber
Cystitis	Blueberries, watermelon, melon, broccoli, strawberries, kiwi fruit, citrus fruit, garlic, yogurt
Depression	Yogurt, egg, lamb, turkey, chicken, seeds and seed oils, fish, greens such as spinach, broccoli, watercress, and kale, parsley, strawberries, kiwi fruit, citrus fruit, oats, quinoa, rye, walnuts, buckwheat
Dermatitis	All fresh fruit and vegetables, especially berries, carrot, sweet pepper, apricot, broccoli, watercress, avocado, mango, pumpkin, and sweet potato, almonds, ginger, garlic, seeds and seed oils, fish
Diabetes	All fruit and vegetable fiber, oats, rye, brown rice, beans, lentils, greens such as spinach, broccoli, watercress, and kale, parsley, yogurt, egg, turkey, chicken, seeds and seed oils, fish
Diarrhea	Apple, carrot, celery (all cooked), white rice, plenty of water, yogurt
Diverticulitis	All fruit and vegetable fiber, oats, rye, brown rice, beans, lentils, yogurt, garlic, ginger, seed oils, fish, papaya, pineapple, cardamom
Dry skin	Berries, watermelon, melon, broccoli, kiwi fruit, garlic, carrot, sweet pepper, watercress, apricot, papaya, avocado, mango, walnuts, almonds, seeds and seed oils, fish
Ear infection	Blueberries, broccoli, strawberries, kiwi fruit, citrus fruit, garlic, onion, ginger, sweet potato, carrot, sweet pepper, apricot, watercress, kale, seeds and seed oils, fish

Eczema	Berries, cherries, carrot, sweet pepper, apricot, broccoli, watercress, avocado, mango, almonds, pumpkin, sweet potato, ginger, garlic, seeds and seed oils, fish, turmeric, walnuts, Brazil nuts, prunes
Fatigue	Sweet potato, pumpkin, banana, spinach, coconut, Jerusalem artichoke, honey, molasses, yogurt, egg, turkey, chicken, seeds and seed oils, fish, lamb, seaweed, buckwheat
Fever	Fresh fruit and vegetable juices, blueberries, broccoli, strawberries, kiwi fruit, citrus fruit, garlic, carrot, sweet pepper, apricot, watercress, kale
Fibroids	All fruit and vegetable fiber, oats, rye, brown rice, beans, lentils, greens such as spinach, broccoli, watercress, and kale, parsley, soy, seeds and seed oils, seaweed, celery
Gall-bladder disorders	Apple, grapefruit, beets, dandelion, yogurt, watercress, cardamom, kale, broccoli
Hemorrhoids	All fruit and vegetable fiber, oats, rye, brown rice, beans, lentils, blueberries, broccoli, strawberries, kiwi fruit, citrus fruit, buckwheat
Hangovers	Carrot, celery, apple, ginger, spinach, broccoli, watercress, kale, parsley, yogurt, garlic, onion, cardamom, pineapple, artichoke, cucumber
Hay fever	All fresh fruit and vegetables, especially blueberries, cherries, carrot, sweet pepper, apricot, broccoli, and watercress, ginger, garlic, seeds and seed oils, fish
Heartburn	Pineapple, papaya, cabbage, dandelion, cardamom, ginger
Herpes	Watermelon, melon, blueberries, strawberries, cherries, carrot, sweet potato, broccoli, kiwi fruit, citrus fruit, avocado, garlic, yogurt

High blood pressure	All fruit and vegetable fiber, oats, rye, brown rice, beans, lentils, broccoli, strawberries, kiwi fruit, citrus fruit, seeds and seed oils, fish, celery, cucumber, garlic, grapes, cinnamon
Hypothyroid	Seaweed, seeds and seed oils, fish
Indigestion	Pineapple, papaya, cabbage, ginger, cardamom
Irritable bowel syndrome	Pineapple, papaya, cabbage, dandelion, fresh vegetable juices, spinach, broccoli, watercress, kale, parsley, yogurt, garlic, onion, ginger, cardamom, pineapple, artichoke, celery, cucumber
Memory problems	Seeds and seed oils, fish, thyme, egg, strawberries, blueberries, watermelon, melon, broccoli, kiwi fruit, citrus fruit, turmeric, walnuts
Menopause-related problems	All fruit and vegetable fiber, oats, rye, brown rice, beans, lentils, greens such as spinach, broccoli, watercress, and kale, parsley, soy, seeds and seed oils, seaweed, celery
Muscle cramps	Spinach, broccoli, watercress, kale, parsley, yogurt, garlic, molasses, seeds, buckwheat
Osteoporosis	Spinach, broccoli, watercress, kale, parsley, yogurt, garlic, molasses, seeds, buckwheat
Premenstrual syndrome	All fruit and vegetable fiber, oats, rye, brown rice, beans, lentils, greens such as spinach, broccoli, watercress, and kale, parsley, soy, seeds and seed oils, seaweed, celery
Prostate problems	Tomato, pumpkin seeds, all fruit and vegetable fiber, oats, rye, brown rice, beans, lentils, greens such as spinach, broccoli, watercress, and kale, parsley, soy, seeds and seed oils, celery

Psoriasis	*Berries, cherries, carrot, sweet pepper, broccoli, watercress, avocado, apricot, almonds, mango, pumpkin, sweet potato, ginger, garlic, seeds and seed oils, fish, turmeric, walnuts, Brazil nuts, prunes*
Sinusitis	*All fresh fruit and vegetables, especially blueberries, strawberries, carrot, apricot, broccoli, watercress, kiwi fruit, pineapple, and onion, ginger, garlic, seeds and seed oils, fish*
Sleeping problems	*Spinach, broccoli, watercress, kale, parsley, yogurt, seeds, buckwheat, banana*
Sprains, strains & other injuries	*Spinach, broccoli, watercress, kale, parsley, cherries, pineapple, papaya, seeds and seed oils, garlic, molasses, turmeric, ginger*
Stress	*Yogurt, egg, lamb, turkey, chicken, seeds and seed oils, fish, spinach, broccoli, watercress, kale, parsley, strawberries, kiwi fruit, citrus fruit, oats, quinoa, rye*
Tonsillitis	*Broccoli, blueberries, strawberries, cherries, kiwi fruit, citrus fruit, garlic, onion, ginger, sweet potato, carrot, sweet pepper, apricot, watercress, kale, seeds and seed oils, fish*
Varicose veins	*All fruit and vegetable fiber, oats, rye, brown rice, beans, lentils, blueberries, strawberries, cherries, kiwi fruit, citrus fruit, broccoli, seeds and seed oils, fish, garlic, ginger, buckwheat, turmeric, prunes, herbs*

wonderfoods glossary

amino acid The building blocks of proteins in our food and throughout the body.

anthocyanidins Powerful antioxidant chemicals found in some plants, particularly blue, red, and purple ones.

antihistamine A substance that counteracts the action of the inflammatory, allergic body chemical histamine.

antioxidant A substance or enzyme that neutralizes oxidants, or free radicals, protecting cells from damage that can lead to disease and aging.

bacteria Minute, single-celled organisms that live in us and in the environment. Some are harmful and others are beneficial.

bile Fluid produced by the liver to help digestion, particularly of fats, and the elimination of waste products.

bioflavonoids Antioxidant chemicals found in some foods.

cardiovascular disease An umbrella term for a range of conditions affecting the heart and blood vessels, such as high blood pressure, atherosclerosis (hardening of the arteries), and high cholesterol.

carotenoids A family of colorful compounds found in foods with antioxidant properties that are considered to be plant forms of vitamin A.

chlorophyll The green pigment in plants, which they need to capture sunlight in order to produce energy.

cholesterol A fat-like substance found in some foods, produced in the liver and present throughout the human body. It's needed in the body, in cell structure for example, and for making some hormones. In excess, it can be a harmful component of cardiovascular disease, particularly when oxidized.

complex carbohydrate Starches and fiber in foods that have not been refined; the starches can be broken down to produce energy.

detoxification The body's natural "cleansing" processes by which it clears waste products and eliminates them.

diuretic A substance that increases the rate of urination, promoting loss of water from the body.

enzyme A protein that acts as a catalyst in any of the countless processes in the body. The term is also used to describe substances that help the breakdown of foods in the gut.

essential fatty acids (EFAs) Fats, such as those found in fish, nuts, and seeds, that are a necessary part of our diet for good health.

fiber A part of foods, especially fruit, vegetables, and whole grains, that the human gut cannot digest. Fiber helps slow down the release of digested food as glucose into the bloodstream, bulks out the stool, feeds beneficial bacteria, and encourages the elimination of waste products.

flavonoids A family of antioxidant chemicals found in some plants.

free radical An oxidant, an atom that is unstable and stabilizes itself by robbing a nearby molecule, thereby creating a cascade of oxidative damage. This process is a normal part of cell workings, but in excess is linked to aging, heart disease, cancer, and other chronic diseases.

fructo-oligo-saccharides (FOS) Indigestible, sweet-tasting, soluble fiber found in some foods, which can be used as fuel by the beneficial bacteria in our intestines.

GLA (gamma linoleic acid) A fatty acid needed for healthy hormone balance, to help lower inflammation and to reduce blood clotting. GLA is found in some plants (borage, for example) and in evening primrose oil. It can also be made in the body as a derivative from linoleic acid (found in seeds such as sunflower).

glucosinolates Chemicals naturally found in some foods, especially the brassica family (broccoli, cabbage, kale, etc.), which help the liver's detoxification processes and act as antioxidants.

harissa This is a North African spice paste. If unobtainable, use a sprinkling of paprika and a dash of hot pepper sauce instead.

hormone Produced in a gland, this is a chemical messenger that travels via blood to sites elsewhere in the body to transmit its specific "message" to cells. Examples are thyroxine (regulates growth and metabolism) and estrogen (the female sex and reproduction hormone).

immune system The body's complex collection of means for protecting against harmful organisms and fighting them once they are in the body.

insulin The hormone produced by the pancreas whose most important role is to help sugar (glucose) get into cells to make energy.

isoflavones Chemicals found in some plants, such as soy, that can have estrogen-like effects in the body.

medium chain triglycerides (MCTs) Fats found in some foods, such as coconut, that are easily absorbed and used to make energy, and appear to help boost metabolism.

mineral Natural inorganic substance, such as iron and magnesium, also called metal. Minerals are found in the earth, in food, and in our bodies, where they form part of the structure and function.

miso A Japanese, fermented soy paste used to make soups.

monounsaturated fats A type of fat, such as that found in olive oil, which has a chemical structure that makes it useful in the body and is linked to good health.

mucous membrane The lubricated lining of passages in the body that open up to the "outside world," i.e. the digestive tract, vagina, and respiratory system.

neurotransmitter A chemical messenger molecule used in the nervous system to convey messages, such as those for memory or mood, between one cell and another.

omega-3 fats A family of fats (found in oily fish, flax seeds, and walnuts, for example) essential for healthy skin, brain, nerves, hormones, and cardiovascular health, as well as lowering inflammation.

omega-6 fats A family of fats (found in sunflower and pumpkin seeds, for example) that are needed in the body for healthy skin and hormones and for lowering inflammation.

oxidant A naturally occurring, unstable molecule that, if left unchecked by sufficient antioxidants, can cause damage to cells. Also known as a free radical.

pectin A type of soluble fiber that is found in some fruits, such as apples, pears, and citrus fruit.

prebiotic Fiber, such as that found in Jerusalem artichokes, that is useful for feeding the beneficial bacteria in the gut.

probiotic A term used to describe beneficial bacteria that we can get from "live" yogurt or in a capsule, which replenishes those we have living in our intestines.

protein Large molecules made up of specific chains of amino acids that are used in and make up the body. They are vital for structure, enzymes, neurotransmitters, and transport in the body.

saturated fat (SF) Fats found in animal-derived foods such as milk, cheese, yogurt, and meat that, in excess, are linked to cardiovascular disease. Coconut and palm oils also contain saturated fat.

serotonin A neurotransmitter made and used in the body, associated with good moods and sleep, among other things.

tahini A paste made from crushed sesame seeds.

tamari A wheatfree sauce made from the fermentation of soybeans, similar to soy sauce.

tryptophan An amino acid that the body can use to make vitamin B3 and serotonin, and needed for growth.

vitamin An organic micronutrient found in foods that is vital to health, normal body processes, and disease prevention.

Index

Acknowledgments

My thanks to...Barbara Levy for always being there, on my team, Anne Furniss with whom
I shared the idea of Wonderfoods over a great salad and a coffee, Jill Mead whose evocative
photography leaves words in the shade, Janet Illsley for expertly knocking my words into
shape, and Ros Holder for making the whole thing look gorgeous. And to my friends who
risked testing recipes: Theresa Banovic, Robert Brennan, Janet Kipling, Marion and Bob Luker.
Also, to my Maltese family cooking greats—Nanna, Auntie Marlene, and Auntie Claire, Arielle
who's not only a fellow piggy but is the best sister ever, and my parents who have always
lavished me with love and good food. And to A, who nourishes my tummy and the rest, not
forgetting my dog Splash, my bees, my computer doctor, and anyone else I've overlooked...